WARDROBE ESSENTIALS
FOR A WOMAN OF *CHARME*

(BLACK AND WHITE EDITION)

Wardrobe Essentials for a Woman of *Charme*

A TIMELESS GUIDE
TO LOOKING SLIM AND CHIC

Chiara Giuliani
with
Benedetta Belloni

ENGLISH EDITION
EDITED BY T. J. CARTER,
ELITE AUTHORS

Text and photographs © 2018 Chiara Giuliani

ISBN: 9781728830056

www.ladonnadicharme.com

DOWNLOAD YOUR
FREE COPY OF THE E-BOOK!
(only for purchases on Amazon.com)

Important Note
to the Black and White
Edition:

The original edition of this book is in full color. We decided to also publish an edition in black and white, to make the book available at a more affordable price. Although the majority of the photos contained in the book are also understandable in black and white, not all of them are. Therefore, for a better understanding of the content, **we recommend downloading your <u>free</u> copy of the e-book on your tablet or PC** (for those who buy the paperback on Amazon.com, the e-book is free of charge) and view it with Kindle Cloud Reader (it's free and easy to use) **in order to view the images in full color.** Furthermore, depending on the chosen device, the photos displayed may appear smaller than the originals; to fix this issue, it is sufficient to <u>click</u> or <u>double-tap on each image</u> <u>to view it on full screen</u>.

Table of Contents

Preface

A few weeks ago, I was walking in the narrow streets of my town, Florence, when I happened to meet a friend of mine whom I have always admired for her class and style and for always being chic and put together. On that day my friend was wearing a mustard-yellow overcoat from a cheap department store—a garment that, due to its color (which is one of the latest trends as I write), certainly did not go unnoticed.

Funny thing—just a few days before, I had seen exactly the same item worn by another woman. The effect, though, was totally different on the two ladies. My friend was chic, trendy, and fashionable. The other woman, conversely, looked frumpy and dowdy.

Yet the "main garment" (the mustard overcoat) was exactly the same: What was the reason for such a stunning difference?

Maybe it was because my friend is a slender girl in her twenties, and the other woman was ninety years old and 250 pounds? No, the two women were more or less the same age and size.

Maybe my chic friend wore expensive designer clothes, whereas the other wore cheap items? Again, this was not the case: conversely, my friend wore garments certainly less expensive than the other's.

The difference consisted merely of different pairings with the other garments.

My stylish friend wore her up-to-the-minute mustard overcoat over a set of staple pieces that suited her body type and made that inexpensive coat look like a designer garment.

The other woman paired the same item with clothes that were certainly trendy but not appropriate to her body and not wisely paired. As a result, she looked like she had taken anything "fashionable" from her closet and thrown it on herself.

This anecdote makes it clear that **if you want to achieve an impeccable style**—a style that calls your name and reflects your inner femininity—**it should be founded on (and supported by) foundation pieces that never go out of style**.

A closet that mainly consists of **versatile, baseline classics perfect for your body shape** and chosen in your signature color palette **allows you to also play around with the most whimsical pieces of the latest trend** while remaining chic and sophisticated.

These garments will allow you to put together polished and stylish outfits in seconds while still keeping to a budget and achieving **a look that will always be trendy**.

Versatile, interchangeable clothing pieces are **perfect for dressing up or down**, depending on the chosen accessories, and they will all look good on you, allowing you to **easily enhance your silhouette**.

These essentials—as the name implies—should form the basis of your wardrobe, but this does *not* mean your closet should only contain baseline staples, because wardrobe essentials allow you to play with the "*non*-staples" in a totally safe way. They allow you to wear even the most up-to-the-minute items without making your outfit look like a cheap mix of mass products (which any chic lady dislikes). And they allow you to achieve a timeless *charme*.

But - you may ask - what does *charme* mean?

Charme is a **French word** whose meaning is slightly different from the English word *charm* and indicates "**an ensemble of beauty, elegance, appeal, allure, and style**."

If you want to get a breathtaking look, if you want people to remember you as charming, chic, and attractive women, you simply have to find out what suits you more. Even the simplest pair of jeans can produce breathtaking results as long as it's in character with your style, body shape and femininity. **You don't**

need to buy countless clothes to achieve this result. You just need to have your perfect baseline staples, those that call your name and flatter your body and personality in a unique (and stylish) way.

This approach to your wardrobe will allow you to **save time and money** and **declutter your closet—and your whole life as well**.

Don't get lost in a chock-full closet and say you have nothing to wear (then run out and buy the twentieth sweater in a color that's up to date but inappropriate for your skin tone). Instead, stock your closet with **perfect, well-established garments** that will allow you to create an easygoing yet chic ensemble that can be easily turned into a more elegant one simply by changing your shoes or by adding a silk scarf. You'll be able to **zero in on what lights you up and focus on quality, thus making an impeccable choice** (that won't be necessarily the most expensive option).

In this book—which further explores some of the topics covered in my previous books, *How to Become a Woman of Charme* and *101 Ways to Look Slimmer and Taller*—we will see, season by season, **the main items you need to build your perfect capsule wardrobe**.

We will also talk about "faux staples": garments usually considered must-haves that are very difficult to wear flawlessly and tastefully combine with other pieces.

The suggestions in this book are supported by pictures that show ensembles that flatter the silhouette—slimming your figure and elongating your legs with the help of simple "geometric" features—as well as combinations that are better to avoid.

With help from this book's tips and pictures, you can achieve **a polished yet easygoing look,** which in addition to making you feel feminine, attractive, and chic, **will boost your self-confidence, enhance your style, and increase your *charme*.**

PART 1

10 Wardrobe Essentials for Summer Clothing

Wardrobe Essentials for Summer Clothing

One of the first things to say about summer clothing is that it's easy to get flawless results. This is partly due to the fact that **deep necklines and bare shoulders and arms** create a kind of **filter area that allows you to play around** with patterns that would otherwise not be so easy to wear. Furthermore, bare legs and arms **always have a slimming effect** on the whole figure.

In addition, **light-colored garments** (white especially) can **flatter your figure while lengthening your body**. When you get tanned (even if only slightly), wearing white or light-colored items can slim your silhouette. The stark contrast of a timeless white dress against dark or tan skin, for example, can make your legs and whole figure look comparatively slimmer and more elongated.

Aside from being a timeless classic suitable for every age, style, and body type, in summer an all-white outfit may also help you look thinner, making this color **one of the staples of slimming summer clothing**—a color that above all is suitable for many different combinations.

With light-colored (but not white) garments, conversely, it's important to be quite careful with pairings. This is particularly true with beige, which—though quite similar to white in tone—is not that similar when it comes to pairing with other colors.

The main difference lies in the fact that beige—which is considered the neutral hue par excellence—should be matched only with other neutral shades. When you pair it with bold, brilliant colors, the outcome is not that brilliant. However, **all lively and vivid colors go well with white, as do neutral**

colors, and for this reason, white can indeed be considered the ultimate summer color.

There is another key aspect to bright colors that is connected to your age: the fuchsia top that looked so cute on you at eighteen can start turning dowdy at thirty-five (even if you are still the same weight). **When you're no longer in your twenties, bold colors worn close to the face can have an unflattering result** because they highlight dark circles and wrinkles. For this reason, it's better to **gradually soften your tones** as you age—even when dressing for summer, when necklines and tanning would seem to allow every color variation. The electric blue of your twenties, for example, can turn into an interesting navy blue when you're forty and change to indigo after sixty. **If you love bright, vibrant colors**, you can **make extensive use of them for your accessories** (shoes and bags above all) regardless of your age.

On the other hand, a totally fashionable pairing—timeless and always stylish whatever your age, style, and body type—is a combination of **black and white** for both garments and accessories. As famous German fashion designer Karl Lagerfeld says, "Black and white always look modern, whatever that word means." This combination always **ensures a polished, put-together, chic, and sophisticated look.** Keep this mind when choosing your outfit, and you will find combinations that enhance your style and personality and are suitable for any setting.

1. White T-Shirt

In the summer months, one of the main staple pieces in every woman's wardrobe is the white T-shirt.

This garment is practical and easy to wear in summer as well as spring and autumn. It allows you to approach every occasion with style and **lends itself to infinite pairings**. It's perfect worn alone or paired with a jacket when it's cooler, allowing you to adapt your look to temperature changes by simply taking off your blazer.

You can find many different patterns in stores and boutiques, making it easy to find a design that **enhances your shape**. The good news is that—unlike what happens with a white shirt—a T-shirt **can also be purchased in cheaper stores with lovely results** thanks to its easy fit. Unlike bold and dark colors, white always delivers impeccable results—even with inexpensive garments.

The drawback is that white, though extraordinary in its versatility and ability to **elevate your look in an instant**, always requires perfectly groomed skin and hair—this is particularly true of white shirts with sleeves and high necklines. A stark white fabric can highlight spots, dark circles, and wrinkles. When buying your staple white T-shirt, **choose low-cut patterns**. A low neckline (even if not *that* low) is generally suitable for all figures, whereas **the classic crew-neck T-shirt isn't good for everyone** because it makes the neck look tougher and enlarges your figure. You should therefore avoid it if you want to look slimmer.

Here some tips for a faultless choice:

(1) The ideal neckline, which enhances every body type, is intermediate: not overhanging nor very low necked.
(2) A **boat neckline** is suitable if you want to look slimmer, because its wide cut **makes your neck look comparatively thinner**.
(3) To get a visually slimmer silhouette, go for **sleeveless patterns** (a sleeveless keyhole top is also very suitable for curvy figures).

(4) If you don't feel comfortable with a low neckline, you can **pair a low-cut T-shirt with a soft linen shirt worn open over your tee**, as we will explain in detail in chapter 4: this way the neckline doesn't draw too much attention while maintaining all its advantages.

(5) The classic **polo shirt** is indeed a timeless pattern, but for those who would like to look slimmer, it's better to **choose a feminine design** with a low neckline and a close-fitting shape that remains close to the body without being too formfitting. Avoid straight designs with the classic three-button neckline, which are suitable only for those who are tall or very thin.

On the subject of fabrics, nice alternatives to the timeless cotton tee include silk (real or synthetic) and linen.

The main characteristic that makes this garment look chic is its color: **when the fabric starts turning gray** (even slightly) or yellowish, and its pristine shiny tone fades, **all its allure goes out the window**. Declutter your wardrobe: be objective and critical and throw away without hesitation any garment that is not totally spotless. You can find new ones at totally reasonable prices— don't think twice and substitute them: you may find new patterns that enhance your figure much more than your old ones. These days it's very easy to find cute patterns and nice fabrics on a budget.

Here are some pairings that can ensure a **polished and sophisticated look**—even with inexpensive garments:

(1) White T-shirt and white capris (or shorts): a definite classic for summertime and vacations. You can brighten this look up with a nice belt for any informal settings.

(2) White T-shirt with straight jeans and low-heeled sandals (or light-colored sneakers): this is a perfect and versatile outfit for many informal events, though since these garments are quite widespread, every accessory must be tasteful and well chosen to avoid looking too ordinary.

(3) Silky white T-shirt and black trousers with jewel sandals (or high-heeled strap sandals): flawless outfit for a party or dinner at a fancy place.

(4) Silky white T-shirt and black trousers with flat shoes or ballet flats (instead of sandals): a look that can be suitable for a business meeting or an easygoing occasion (depending on the shoe style).

If you want to look thinner, a white T-shirt is almost **the only option you can combine with light-colored shorts**: in the pictures below, the figure on the right seems much slimmer than the one on the left (wearing a dark-colored polo shirt).

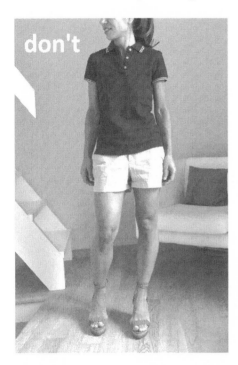 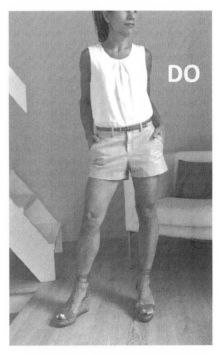

A white T-shirt is also the easiest piece to **pair with a skirt that has an unconventional color or pattern**, as it plays down anything eccentric (be it an accessory, a print, or a shade), making otherwise difficult-to-match garments wearable. Add a nice pair of sandals, and you can look chic and polished (whereas a black T-shirt on the same outfit would look quite dated).

Also, **you can wear your white T-shirt with a skirt that's too sexy** or eye-catching: a classic white tee can tone down the sex appeal, **making you look much more interesting and elegant**.

One last thing: graphic tees have been trendy for some time now. You can easily find them in cheaper stores as well as designer boutiques. Personally, I think **too many prints can turn a stylish, alluring, and versatile garment into something boring and ordinary**. If you want to buy a graphic tee, my suggestion is to spend as little as possible on it. It's just a fad, and it's not worth spending a lot on clothes you won't want to wear in a few months. This way you can keep your style safe as well as your budget.

2. Striped Shirt

Another staple piece for the warm season is the classic striped shirt (also called "Breton shirt"), a must-have garment of the Parisian chic style that's been **worn by many style icons** over time. Traditionally this article belonged to sailors. In the twentieth century, it became a staple of women's fashion thanks to **Coco Chanel** (who used to wear it with red lipstick and pearls), **Marilyn Monroe, Brigitte Bardot**, and many others. This garment has also been worn by artists—even male artists—who have made it their signature uniform (Pablo Picasso and Jean Paul Gaultier).

This clothing piece can make you look effortlessly **chic and classy**; its alternating colors, if paired with the right garment, can easily enhance your face, body, and style.

Unlike the white T-shirt, which focuses attention on your face, the striped shirt **plays down wrinkles, dark circles, and any imperfection**. For this reason, the striped shirt **doesn't require a low neckline (like the white tee does)**, which makes it a simpler choice than a solid-color tee.

The original pattern is white and blue (according to tradition, the white stripes made a sailor who fell into the sea more visible to his buddies), but nowadays there are plenty of colors, patterns, and variations (some of which are **also suitable for city life**). You can have fun experimenting with which combinations are the most suitable to your colors, shape, and style.

Furthermore, this garment is timeless and fashionable not only as a short-sleeved T-shirt but as a long-sleeved one (which was the original design worn by sailors).

A nice striped shirt is a perfect garment for women of all styles and ages. Furthermore, interestingly enough, **a striped shirt whose dominant color matches your pants can lengthen your silhouette in a flattering way.** This is contrary to the common wisdom that horizontal stripes have an enlarging effect, but *it works*, making your figure look more elongated and harmonizing your forms in a very flattering way. A solid-color T-shirt whose color contrasts with pants, on the other hand, isn't very flattering.

But be warned: to produce a slimming effect, **the stripes that match the pants must be wide enough** and should preferably be the dominant color of the tee.

As is crystal clear in the photos below, if you pair white pants with a black-and-white-striped shirt that has very thin white stripes (on the left), it will widen the figure. In the other two images, the effect is slender and very chic.

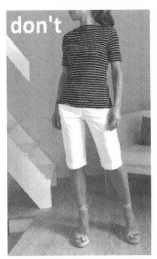 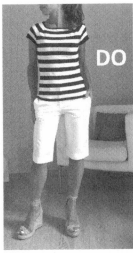 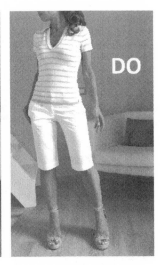

This garment is a must-have in summertime for the whole family—both short sleeved and long sleeved. A fine lightweight cotton shirt is great for the heat, as it caresses your body without being too tight, **protecting your skin while refreshing your body**. It's much more pleasant to wear than a synthetic microfiber tank top, which lends itself to a sweat bath.

This garment is perfect when combined with shorts, jeans, cotton trousers (even those with an elegant cut), and also skinny jeans and heeled sandals.

The striped shirt also allows you to wear dark colors—otherwise not suitable for summer—because the dark tone is lightened by the striped pattern, which makes this item **a stylish and sophisticated piece that maintains an informal feel**.

Pairing black trousers with a black-and-white striped tee and a bright-colored jacket is also totally chic (and suitable for spring as well).

One last tip: when buying this garment, **be sure its cut is continuous**—meaning that the stripes continue on both sides of the seams. If the stripes are visually interrupted, this defect can be seen even from far away, reducing the allure of even the most sought-after look.

I will conclude this chapter by sharing a few words from my coauthor, Benedetta (a big fan of this item):

With a striped shirt, you wear **a garment with a story to tell**—not those of the Breton fishermen or Coco Chanel, but **your story** (even if you have never spent windy summers in the harbors). I remember an important fashion fair in Milan; after a whole day spent among amazing women, I realized that the only one who had really impressed me was a very chic brunette who wore a wonderful silky striped shirt with a pair of blue trousers. Sometimes we try to look different, or we try trendy outfits whose appeal is on a ticking clock; but instead, **we can learn to find our style by starting from simplicity**.

The results, believe me, will be extraordinary!

3. Capri Pants

Capri pants are another classic of the summer wardrobe. It is indeed **a timeless garment** loved by many twentieth-century sex symbols—from Brigitte Bardot to Marilyn Monroe—who gave it **ageless allure and vibrant sensuality**.

Though some believe this item is only suitable for tall and slender women, this is not the case.

The only essential requisite for wearing capri pants flawlessly is having **slender ankles: not *very* thin but visibly thinner than the calf** (a feature that many women have, even if they complain about a few extra pounds around the hips or in the bust area). Furthermore, **highlighting your ankle always has an overall slimming effect**, as it makes your whole figure look leaner.

Conversely, capri pants are not suitable for those who, even if slender, have puffy ankles. For these women, it's better to choose Bermudas that reach the knee and do not highlight the ankles.

If carefully paired, capris can work for many different places and occasions.

Furthermore, **they have the added value of being easy to pair with flat shoes** (ballet flats above all), whereas they don't look so good when paired with high-heeled shoes. This makes them **one of the rare garments that is totally sexy yet practical** and joins comfort and style.

Here are some suggestions for possible pairings:

(1) If you have a strong calf, opt for a slightly longer capri design so that the hem does not come exactly to the middle of the calf but a little bit lower; also remember that you can create a slimming effect on the calf by choosing tones that are lighter than your skin (white is especially good for this).

(2) Capri pants with a striped shirt make a lovely and timeless outfit (for a slimming effect, see the tips mentioned in chapter 2).

(3) Capri pants with ballet flats guarantee a flawless and chic outcome. Conversely, it's better to **avoid pairings with**

strappy sandals, because they can **shorten the part of your leg that remains in plain sight** (as the picture on the left clearly shows).

(4) For the same reason, it's better to avoid high-heeled shoes, because **heels create an extra gap that visually reduces the length of your lower leg,** shortening your figure while enlarging your silhouette (this effect is even more visible from behind).

(5) If you are a heel addict, you can go for sandals with wedges as long as their color is of a similar tone to your skin: wedges visually extend the line of the leg instead of breaking it, as heels may do.

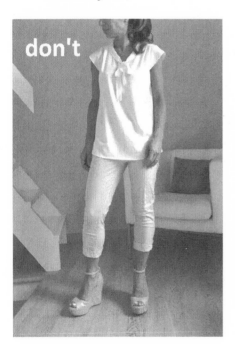 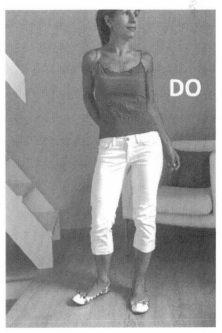

The accompanying top should not be chosen lightly. Since capri pants are so versatile, the top is the key element that defines your style and mood; with a single choice, you characterize your entire look.

If you prefer an informal yet classic style, a cute choice is a simple polo shirt—as long as it's quite formfitting and has a medium neckline that lengthens your figure.

If your goal is a bon ton look, pair capri pants with a shaped boatneck top in a quality fabric that follows your figure and enhances it.

Avoid loose tops and sweaters, which **add unnecessary volume to your figure** (as in the picture on the left). If you don't love formfitting garments, you can overlay an open boyfriend shirt over a low-cut top (as we'll better explain in the next chapter).

When the weather gets cooler, capri pants **can be paired with a straight, lightweight coat** worn open—a classy and chic outfit that is also very appropriate for springtime.

4. Linen Shirt

Another must-have for summer is undeniably the linen shirt (or a lightweight cotton shirt), a garment that is **comfortable, cool, easygoing, and chic** at the same time. It also has the priceless advantage of being **stylish even when lightly wrinkled**, which makes it a wonderful garment for travel, whatever your destination.

Moreover, this is a decidedly multipurpose piece that **can be paired in a thousand different ways** depending on your body, mood, and taste, making it suitable for all styles and many settings.

Don't forget, though, that this item must be **wide and soft**: close-fitting shirts can only be worn when it's cooler, as such shirts worn in the heat can transform even the most sophisticated lady into a Sahara crossing survivor in minutes.

Conversely, **a boyfriend shirt** has an effect similar to that of a parasol for old-time ladies: it **shades your body and keeps you cool**.

You can wear it open or closed over your swimwear or with straight (or capri) pants and a low-cut top, but **avoid any pairings with loose trousers** (unless you are six feet tall) or with minidresses, because these combinations can enlarge your figure, as shown in the image on the left.

Another benefit is that it's possible to find lovely linen shirts at a very reasonable price—unlike the classic shirt we will discuss about later on, which can be quite expensive. Here are a few reasons why linen shirts are so inexpensive:

(1) First of all, linen (or very light cotton) shirts are one of the staples for many cheap brands during the summer.
(2) Secondly, the ideal linen shirt is quite wide (it's an almost unstructured garment), so **it is not necessary to have one tailored**: even a straight and simple cut is suitable (indeed it's the *most* suitable).
(3) You can even **steal this item from your partner's wardrobe** (at no cost at all!) or find it in the kids' department. The main

cheap brands produce this item for boys up to about five feet seven, which means that most of us can get this timeless garment at a very good price.

This item is suitable for all ages and all body types, and it can be worn open over a top or swimsuit. When knotted at the waist and paired with shorts or low-waisted jeans, **it can become a totally sexy item**. It's **also suitable for those who feel more comfortable being covered**—if you pair a linen shirt with capri pants (or jeans) and a low-cut top, you'll end up with a flawless outfit that **helps hide your waist or not-exactly-toned arms**.

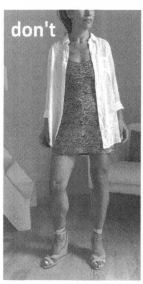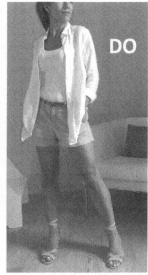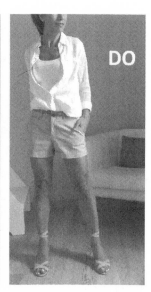

This garment is also perfect for sunny days because **it helps prevent sunburns** and protects your skin much better than a formfitting synthetic top (which will make you melt in the heat).

It's also suitable for a late-afternoon date or an informal dinner.

It can **keep you warm when the autumn winds start blowing** or help you avoid peeling skin from too much sunbathing.

Linen shirts work for traveling, too; during a flight, I once saw a girl with khaki-and-white-striped capri pants, a white top, and an open khaki linen shirt, which created a chic, stylish, and classy look that was comfortable and easygoing.

On cooler evenings you can also **tuck it into your jeans and leave it unbuttoned halfway up**, showing a lace or bright-colored top.

A linen shirt is always practical, fresh, and comfortable. Keep in mind that a long-sleeved shirt will not make you too hot: thanks to its wide line and natural fabric, it shades your skin while protecting you from the heat.

Here are a few suggestions regarding color:

(1) It's preferable to stick to **neutral tones**—from the classic and timeless white to beige, light gray, oatmeal, flax, sand, and the like.
(2) **Avoid dark colors**, which can take any refreshing effect away.
(3) Pastel colors can be pleasant, but they're not easy to pair: choose these hues only if you're sure of the possible combinations.
(4) A **light-colored boyfriend shirt layered over a dark-colored top and trousers** (see the picture on the left in chapter 14) creates a slender, elegant silhouette that **helps hide extra pounds**.

This garment, as mentioned at the beginning, is nice even if slightly wrinkled. When you're on vacation, you can wash it and dry it on a hanger, and it will be **wearable without needing to be ironed**.

You can also wear it in informal city settings, for a trip out of town, or in spring with a pair of jeans, a nice belt, and light-colored sneakers. You can also keep it in your bag when you go to an air-conditioned supermarket on a very hot day.

With this item, you will always have a **lovely, easygoing look** that is also **chic, classy, and inexpensive**. What more could you need?

5. Light-Colored Shorts

Shorts and Bermuda shorts, once worn mainly by the sea or for holidays, have become **suitable for the city**, and this is a very good thing, because they can provide an easygoing look while remaining totally fashionable.

However, it is important to remember that these garments, by their very nature, **still maintain an informal air**; therefore the pairings must be carefully chosen to guarantee a harmonious outcome.

When **pairing with shoes**, for instance, it's better to go **open-toed** (sandals and flip-flops) or informal (ballet flats and light-colored sneakers). Pairing them with pumps could look odd or excessive (and not exactly chic).

As for colors, it's ideal to **choose light colors and use matching tones for your upper and lower body**. This always guarantees a chic look while elongating the figure and **making your legs look longer and slimmer** (conversely, it's better to avoid too-dark hues as well as combinations of contrasting colors between your upper and lower body).

Since white and beige shorts are so common, remember that **white shorts can be paired with tees of any color** (bright, dark, bold, or lively), **whereas the beige ones *can't*.**

This is because **beige**, the "king" of neutral hues, **only goes well with other neutral tones** (white, gray, sand, taupe, or similar—though combinations with black can achieve a city-like effect). Instead, **it's better to avoid any combination of beige and bold colors**. Conversely, you'll get a classy and faultless result if you match white shorts with bright-colored garments.

Shorts in pastel or lively shades may also have lovely results. Since shorts are far from your face, they allow you to **choose tones that aren't totally suitable for your complexion**. You can lighten it up with a low-cut white top and light-colored sandals for a stylish and put-together look (whereas bold-colored tees aren't so flawless when you're no longer in your twenties).

Here are some useful tips to enhance and slim the figure:

(1) For those who don't have long and slender legs, **Bermuda shorts require a wedge, even if minimal**. If you're not one of the tall ladies out there, you'd better pair your Bermuda shorts with cork wedge sandals or choose shorts instead (they make the legs look longer).

(2) If you want to make your leg look thinner and longer, it's fundamental to choose the correct length of shorts and Bermuda shorts. **Midthigh lengths** or Bermudas that end a few inches above the knee are not usually helpful for a short leg (as you can see on the left), as they **can make your thighs look fuller, highlight your knees**, and make your hips and legs look larger than they really are.

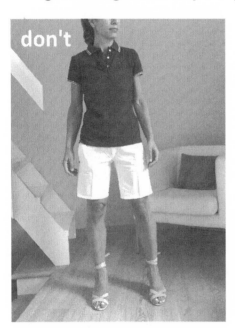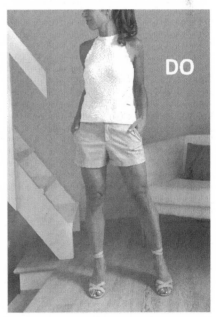

For this reason, it's better to wear Bermudas that arrive exactly at the knee or **otherwise go for shorts**: if you choose shorts that are decidedly short, you'll get a taller and slimmer figure.

As you can see from the comparison between the two pictures, the short shorts (on the right), make **the legs look longer and the figure slimmer** than the figure on the left. The knee, even if uncovered, is not highlighted, and any imperfections can easily pass unnoticed.

Interestingly enough, **shorts can have a slightly less informal look than Bermudas** (which are a more sporty garment). Also, you can wear shorts with ballet flats, flip-flops, or low-heeled sandals with an excellent outcome.

Don't forget that it's preferable to pair light-colored shorts and Bermudas with similarly light-colored tops (be they short-sleeved tees, keyhole tops, polos, or tank tops). As you can see in the pictures, **contrasting colors on your upper and lower body** (on the left) **widens the figure and makes it look fuller**, whereas choosing similar tones (on the right) slims your figure while enhancing your silhouette.

Also, you can get lovely results by pairing shorts with a lightweight long-sleeved shirt—very chic and totally suitable when the weather is not too hot. Conversely, Bermudas with long-sleeved shirts may result a slightly overdressed look.

6. White Dress

A dress, whatever its color, is unquestionably one of the fashion staples for summer. This garment can easily **flatter your body type while enhancing your personal style**. When it's hot, wearing a dress is always an easy choice, because you **don't need to think of any combination**—just decide whether to make it more or less sophisticated with heels or flat shoes, with costume jewelry or your grandma's necklace (the only exception is the sheath dress, which I deem one of the "faux wardrobe essentials").

A dress is a lovely choice for all types of women. It can help you save time in the morning and make you feel graceful and fresh during the day (and also **very feminine**). A dress can give you the feeling of being **polished and cool—stylish but comfortable**.

It's important to note that **a dress can easily hide any imperfections around your waist or on your legs**: a flared medium-length dress can magnificently minimize your buttocks, hips, and thighs (while highlighting your breast, if you want). Even those who find it difficult to hide extra pounds or unpleasant bulges with trousers or a skirt **can feel like Greek goddesses with the appropriate dress**.

Choosing a dress can also bring a refreshing new element to your look: even if you are not used to wearing dresses, you may one day accidentally come across a dress that suits you, helping you reveal your femininity. This could give you the opportunity to **feel more beautiful, feminine, and attractive**, with a new desire to take care of yourself.

If you wear a **white dress** (or a light-colored one), not only will you see **a slimming effect for your whole figure** (as we will see in a while) but you'll also have a **timeless and classy outfit** suitable for many different occasions. The truth is that bright-colored or fancy-printed dresses, even if perfectly cut, can seldom be appropriate for all occasions. Shoes and accessories may help a lot, of course, but a dress of this kind never loses its own character. Also, fancy fabrics for dresses must be carefully chosen, because they can enlarge your figure and make you seem fuller.

Conversely, in the summer, a **white or light-colored dress** is always a chic yet easygoing choice that **can flatter your body while enhancing your style**.

Sleeveless dresses produce the **maximum slimming effect**. Sleeves may have the unpleasant outcome of visually enlarging your whole figure, as you can see in the comparison between the photos below. Therefore, if you want to look thinner, it's better to go for sleeveless patterns. If you are afraid you'll be cold, **you can overlay your dress with a beautiful stole**, which—as we will see in detail in chapter 20—is another staple suitable for everyday life.

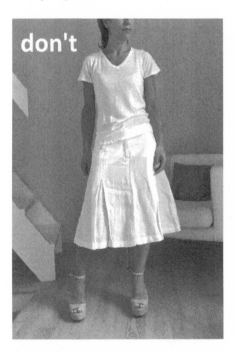 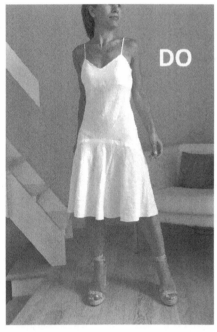

If you find your perfect summer dress, you will get a powerful yet easy tool to **enhance your look and amaze those around you**.

Here some tips on how to wear a light-colored dress flawlessly while hiding a few extra pounds:

(1) For the wide-busted ladies out there, it's essential to choose dresses with a low neckline, which can help slim your silhouette while highlighting your physical assets.

(2) If you have a few extra pounds around your hips and thighs, choose a flared pattern that shapes your upper body and is loose at the bottom. Also, don't forget that a white dress can make your legs look thinner (see above).

(3) If you want to hide a few pounds around your waist and are lucky enough to have lean legs and arms, go for a tunic dress.

(4) **When you are tanned** (even if slightly), **wearing white or light-colored dresses is always flattering**, because—due to the contrasting colors between fabric and skin—your legs will immediately seem thinner. Be aware, though, that **your white dress must *never* be formfitting—otherwise you will highlight what you're trying to hide**.

(5) If you'd like to look taller, it's better to avoid long dresses. If you really want to wear a long dress, balance it out with a deep neckline.

As for the arms, even if they are not exactly thin or toned, they will remain unnoticed if you choose a dress with a medium or low neckline (bare skin always has a slimming effect).

If you have **strong hips but a thin ankle**, you can look good with one of those **deconstructed or trapezoidal midcalf dresses in natural fabrics** (such as linen) paired with leather sandals.

Don't forget that patterns that have a horizontal seam around the hips always widen your hips (even if narrow), so they're only suitable for those who are very thin and want to look fuller.

If you have a wide breast, another suitable and always chic choice is a **wrap dress**, with which you will always look amazing.

It's better to pick out patterns with a simple and classic cut (any of those mentioned before are acceptable). Extravagant or fancy dresses may be gorgeous, but they're not likely to be suitable for many occasions: buy them only if you already have your perfect white dress in your wardrobe.

As for fabrics, in the hot season it's preferable to go for linen, cotton, or a beautiful and lightweight viscose. The results will be magnificent, and your staple dress will make you feel **chic, stylish, attractive, and even comfortable** as a pair of trousers could never do.

7. Wedge Sandals

Wedge sandals are a timeless staple in summer. They're versatile enough to be paired with different outfits and **may be worn in any informal setting** in the city, on the weekend, or when you're on vacation.

The main advantage of wedge sandals is that they **allow you to wear high heels while remaining totally comfortable** to walk on, and they're the perfect shoe option for every woman and every shape because they **circumvent the dilemma of finding the most appropriate heel style for your legs**.

Nevertheless, though this item can be suitable for many pairings and body types, its **informal character** makes it inappropriate for work (where it's better to go for classic pumps) and more formal events (where stiletto sandals—from classic styles to fancy ones—may have a better outcome).

Plus, wedge sandals have an added value appreciated by those who do not feel comfortable with heels: they **allow you to wear shoes with a slight platform** (permitting you to walk easily and safely with a heel that's higher than your usual). Wedge sandals— especially **when they're in cork or rope and have an easygoing style**—are one of the rare shoes that **can sport a platform without looking tasteless** and without making your legs seem shorter than they are (as is frequently the case when you wear platform pumps).

Choosing the appropriate color and shape is essential for a flawless and chic outcome. A wedge can help your legs look longer and slimmer, as it will lengthen your figure while making your silhouette look thinner, but **thick, dark wedges do not necessarily have the same lovely outcome**.

Here some tips for flawless results:

(1) The wedge should **preferably be in rope or cork in its natural color**: these materials visually **stretch your leg** without creating any disproportion between the leg and the heel.

(2) **Dark wedges shorten the legs and widen the figure** (as is clear from the comparison between the pictures below), so it's better to avoid them if you want to look slimmer and more chic.

(3) It's essential that not only the wedge but **also the shoe itself** (the leather or fabric part, to be clear) **be as similar in color as possible to your legs**. As an alternative to the classic nude, you may also get very chic results with colors like yellow, orange, and pink.

(4) Avoid dark colors or hues that contrast with your skin. Be aware that even colors like blue and green, though pretty, should be used with care if you want to achieve a lengthening effect (**if you're lucky enough to have long, lean legs, you can use any color you like**).

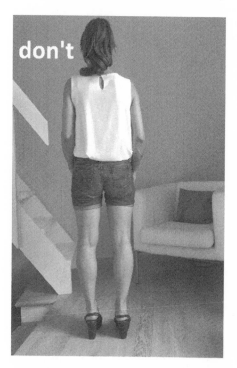 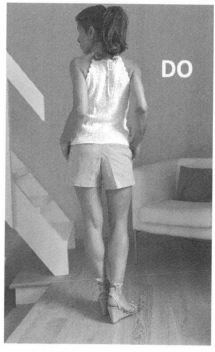

The shoe style should preferably be minimal in order to take advantage of the slimming effect of the bare skin. If the shoe covers the main part of your foot, your legs will look fuller, highlighting any imperfections.

If you choose a style with straps, the **ankle strap** should be fastened around the thinner part of your ankle—*above* **the malleolus, not** *under* **it**. A strap fastened lower (where the ankle is wider) shifts the attention toward the wider part of your ankle and has the effect of making your ankle and leg appear fuller, shortening your leg.

If your foot is not exactly tiny, instead of using nude hues (which can elongate your leg but have the drawback of making your feet look bigger), you may use **colors that slightly contrast with your skin but still have a lighter tone**: white, gray, yellow, orange—even red if the design is really minimalist. When used for shoes that have a minimalist pattern, these colors can **make your feet look more elegant and sexy**; they draw the attention toward the shoe and **away from imperfections in your feet, thus enhancing your sex appeal**.

8. Ballet Flats

Ballet flats are another perfect statement piece that never goes out of style—an item that lends itself to many different pairings and can be worn by women of all ages and body types. Though this type of shoe has little or no heel, **it can make your figure look proportional and even slender** if carefully paired, thanks to two key elements:

(1) As ballet flats leave your foot mostly uncovered, you can benefit from the **slimming effect of naked skin** (without the drawback of making your feet look bigger, as some medium-heeled shoes do).

(2) Furthermore, interestingly enough, since they have little or no heel, **ballet flats can make your legs appear longer. High heels**, though they add inches to your height, **may create an extra breakpoint** that can reduce the visual length of your lower leg, while of course this doesn't happen with ballet flats.

Keep in mind that, if you want to achieve a slimming effect and get a chic and polished look, you do not necessarily have to always resort to very high heels. **You can achieve an amazing outcome by simply choosing those shoes most suitable for your body type**, enhancing your figure while making it proportional. Ballet flats can help you achieve this result easily.

A five-inch heel, if it's not suited to the shape and length of your legs, can make you look full bodied while increasing the circumference of your legs (this is particularly true for platform shoes, which do not look good on most women, as we will see in chapter 35). Conversely, **a lower and comfortable heel**, if carefully chosen, **can indeed make you look much more stylish and even slender**.

Still, don't forget that—though it's absolutely unfair—if you're one of the tall ladies out there, you can go for whatever heel height you prefer. Conversely, if you're shorter than average, you should never overdo the height of your heel; otherwise the heel can seem longer than your calf.

Ballet flats instantly bypass all those heel issues, and for this reason, they are one of the most suitable shoe types for a timeless, classy, and chic look.

As mentioned in the previous chapters, **many summer trousers create a lovely outcome when paired with ballet flats**.

If you match a pair of ballet flats with shorts or capri pants, the leg looks harmonious and proportional (as you can see below on the right and in the middle), whereas heels should be avoided because they can weigh down your figure, highlighting any imperfections.

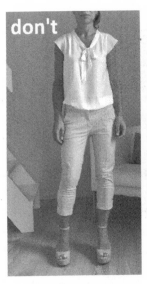 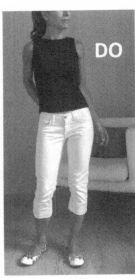 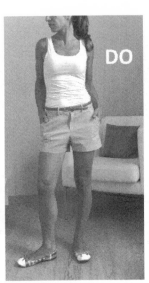

As mentioned above and in chapters 3 and 5, ballet flats always go perfectly with

(1) capri pants, because they work with ballet flats to visually extend the leg line (unlike what a pair of sneakers would do) and do not create an extra breakpoint in your lower leg (as a higher heel would do);

(2) straight pants, as long as the hem is short enough to leave your ankle uncovered; and

(3) shorts, because even in this case, your leg is visually lengthened.

Since ballet flats cover your toe, **they make your feet look shorter and your legs longer by contrast**, as you can see in the picture on the right.

Nonetheless, **ballet flats are not suitable for pairings with long, wide-leg pants or with Bermudas**, which usually require a minimal heel (unless you have very thin and long legs).

Be aware, though, that when combining ballet flats with pants, **it is essential to adjust the hem to the right height** (as explained in detail in chapter 11). If you don't hem your pants properly, leaving them wrapped like ivy around your ankles, the outcome is not slimming or chic. If you hem your pants at the correct height—so that they gently follow your legs, shaping them without being too tight or messy,—you get a polished and stylish look, which will help you appear thinner.

As for the style of the shoe itself, the **cap toe** or **bicolor** (where the toe has a different color than the rest of the shoe) is **an ageless classic** that—as Madame Chanel teaches—**enhances your foot, making it look more proportional**.

A **metal buckle** can be lovely, feminine, and polished, and it **can add a touch of formality**.

If you do not have long, thin legs, you should avoid ankle straps attached to low-heeled shoes, as the straps will divide your lower leg and enlarge your figure instead of highlighting a thin ankle.

If you can't imagine wearing no-heel shoes, you can opt for a little heel but keep it quite low (maximum one inch); otherwise the chic, timeless effect is lost.

As for color, **nude hues** may not be the best choice for ballet flats. They **can make your feet look bigger and longer** and are therefore only suitable for those with tiny feet. Those with larger feet should **go for light colors as well as bright** ones: the warmer and lighter hues are suitable for slimming, whereas the cold ones are more suitable for those with long (or thin) legs.

9. Leather Belt

Another foundation piece in the summer months is undoubtedly a belt (be it leather or another material), which, if carefully chosen and paired, can **customize your outfit** and **enhance your silhouette**.

A belt can look flattering not only for those looking to highlight a thin waistline but **also for those who would like to camouflage a few extra pounds**.

If worn slightly higher than the actual waist, a belt can slim your figure, **drawing attention to itself and away from your hips or thighs**.

Furthermore, a belt can help you achieve an hourglass shape, which always has a slimming effect.

Wide garments can make your figure look more full-bodied, whereas **a belt gives your clothes a shaped form in the middle, allowing you to leave the rest of your garments as loose as you prefer**, which helps to hide what you want to hide.

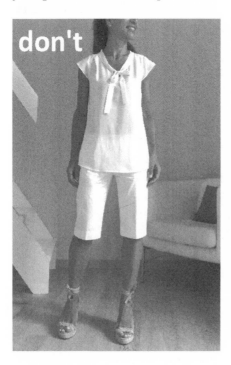
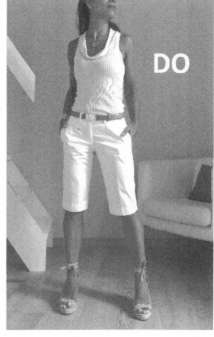

Adding a belt over a knee-length dress is essential for those who are quite short-statured: a dress that looks formless without a belt becomes chic and feminine with a belt.

Moreover, pairing a nice belt with a wide, medium-length skirt makes the lower part of the skirt appear wider, while the legs and waist look comparatively slimmer.

The belt **is also a must when wearing trousers that are too loose around your waist**. Many women, even if they may have a few extra pounds around the hips, have a rather narrow waistline. In this case, wearing a belt is essential because trousers that are too loose on your waist enlarge your whole figure. Wearing a belt allows you to choose the most suitable size for the hip area, removing any excessive looseness around your waist.

Be aware, though, that wearing a belt may not be the most flattering choice if you don't have a proportionate waistline (which *doesn't* mean a *thin* one, but a waistline that's visibly thinner than your hips and breast). In this case a belt should be worn very carefully; **if there is not enough contrast between your waist and your upper and lower body**, the figure may look less feminine, while the bust may look boxy, so **it's better to avoid belts** and choose garments that remain loose on the bust instead of highlighting it.

Conversely, **a belt is perfect for curvy body types because it helps shape your silhouette, adding a sexy and feminine touch** to your look.

Here are some tips to help you achieve the most flattering outcome:

(1) It's best to go with clean, flat styles (without too many decorative elements) and a smooth, simple buckle.
(2) The **buckle** itself should never be underestimated: **a metal one** is usually the easier and most flattering choice (as long as it's quite small) since adding something small and bright at waist height is always nice, and it helps to slim your figure.
(3) **The buckle should never be too big or too flashy**, however, otherwise the effect will be exactly the opposite.
(4) Also avoid plastic buckles (they can make even the most polished outfit appear ordinary) as well as those with some

famous huge logo: far from upgrading your look, they do just the opposite.

When it comes to pairing with shoes or bags, the choice depends on the colors of the belt itself. **Wearing a leather belt and camel shoes is a chic and timeless choice**, but pairing a bright-turquoise belt with bright-turquoise shoes can be excessive and not exactly tasteful. A flashy belt visually divides your figure (this is not the case for shoes, which can be brightly colored and still enhance your figure, as - it goes without saying - they do not stay around your midsection).

For this reason, it's better to stay on the safe side and **give preference to neutral shades, be they light and dark** or even **deep ones** if you want, while **avoiding bold, lively ones** (which means choosing a deep wine hue instead of simply red and mustard instead of bright yellow). Contrasting colors in your midsection are not the best if you want to look slender, whereas **neutral shades always help give continuity to your figure, making it look slimmer**.

You can have fun playing with slightly lighter or darker shades (for example, white sandals can be paired with a light gray belt), though don't forget that **the leather belt is a summer staple** (in all shades of natural leather). This tonality can be worn with almost any garment, becoming **a real statement piece** for summer. A leather belt can help simplify your outfit choices, while giving you **a polished and chic look**. It's also great for travel as it lends itself to countless possible combinations without taking up much space in your luggage, and is **perfect for all garments and all occasions.**

10. Leather Bag

Bags are unquestionably one of the key statement pieces in every woman's look; beyond that, they are considered iconic items. In addition to its pure practicality, **a bag is often perceived as an extension of ourselves**. It's no coincidence that some bags—or to be more precise, some designer handbags—are often **considered an easy way to feel stylish, tasteful, and à la page**, representing a sort of status symbol that can effortlessly open doors to the world of luxury and glamour.

Believe me, this is not always the case. As my co-author (and cousin) Benedetta cleverly points out,

> If the bag you are carrying is one of those plastic models with an unmistakable signature all over its surface, not only is it not worth a tenth of its price, but it also takes any class and elegance away. This type of product is undeniably a mass product, created for a clientele which is supposed to be quite ordinary, so if you want to be remembered as a chic, elegant, classy, and attractive lady—and not just like that chick with the designer handbag—then go for something different, and you will gain in class and personality.

Now let's talk about how to choose the right bag.

The first thing to keep in mind is that **if you want to have a chic and sophisticated look**, then your bag should preferably be **leather** (or at least **canvas**, as long as its material is high quality). Of course, you may still have some plastic shoulder bags for the beach or very casual dates, but they should *not* be your main ones.

Here are a few tips for a flawless choice:

1. The material must be or stiff or very soft: any in-betweens have a dowdy and unsatisfactory look.
2. It's essential that **metal details**—if present—are **high quality**: they must be **spotless, faultless, and sparkling**. Metal details make the quality of an item unmistakable; you may carry a cheap handbag yet look just as good if you make a

tasteful choice and if the bag itself doesn't have any metal details. But if you want to buy an item with some metal parts, then go for quality items.

3. **Handles often get damaged**—to prevent this, you can **tie a small scarf around them**, which may also be a stylish and feminine touch that can elevate your outfit.

A bag may be used as a key element that **can boost any outfit (even the most easygoing one)**, making your look unique and classy. A bright-colored bag, for instance, can brighten a dark outfit or an outfit mainly composed of interchangeable baseline garments (such as blue jeans and a white shirt), adding a note of color while enhancing your style.

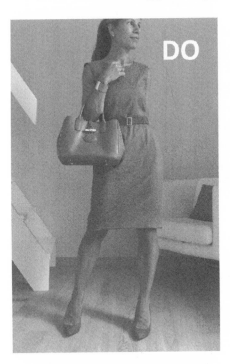
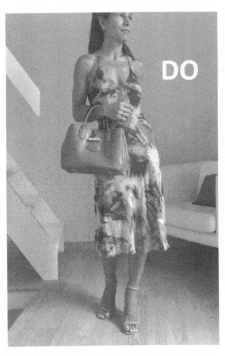

It must be said that **in the summer months, the real foundation piece**—a piece that never goes out of style whatever the trends say about colors and is the perfect option for any setting—is a **leather bag in its natural color** (be it tan, caramel, camel, or lighter). As you can see in the photos above, a **natural leather**

bag strikes a **perfect balance between casual and sophisticated**, and it's versatile enough to be paired with many outfits, from shorts to midcalf dresses.

If you find the one bag that calls your name, you'll have found the perfect item for warmer months (it may also be appropriate in winter, if you want), and **you can bring it on any trip or vacation with no need to carry another bag**. (And you won't have to pay any extra fee for your next flight!)

As with a leather belt, you can't go wrong with a bag in this hue, because it helps you look slimmer, hiding any extra volume around your waist, and besides, it really goes with everything.

Summer **pastel colors**, though lovely, may not be the easiest choice. If you don't carefully match your pastel bag with your other garments, the outcome can be a color palette that maybe is artistically striking in itself but can result inappropriate if your goal is to achieve a chic and sophisticated look (though pastel colors are very **helpful for livening up an all-dark look in the winter**).

With regard to the purchase of a new item, though from where I live (Florence, Italy), I could say it's quite easy to find high-quality, low-priced leather bags, I'm aware this is not the case in other countries. My suggestion is to **browse online shops** (you can find many top quality brands based not only in Italy but in France as well. Furthermore, if you take a peek to our blog from time to time, you may find helpful tips to shopping online with a totally satisfying outcome). Love the thrill of the chase—it may reveal exciting and fun, and it will allow you to discover **small brands (or even family-run businesses) that produce amazing leather at the most affordable prices**. This may require some time and patience, but you'll come across fine handmade products whose quality is equal to, if not higher than, world-famous brands.

In this way, **you** (and not just another signature yet ordinary bag) - **will be in the spotlight with your unique personality and allure,** to the benefit of your style and *charme*!

PART 2

10 Wardrobe Essentials for Spring and Autumn Clothing

Wardrobe Essentials
for Spring and Autumn Clothing

Most wardrobe staples change depending on the season. This is not just because some garments are totally different from the warmer months to the cooler months (no one wears a cashmere turtleneck in the summer) but also because **a given combination produces a different outcome from season to season.**

For example, in winter you can wear almost any kind of skirt thanks to the fact that—when paired with a dark turtleneck, dark opaque stockings, and dark shoes—the skirt flatters your silhouette making it look more proportional, whereas in autumn and spring the same ensemble would look overdressed. Similarly, **a dress**—which in summer is one of the main statement pieces— **is not that easy to wear flawlessly in other seasons.** A lightweight, sleeveless flared dress can be suitable for different settings simply by changing your accessories (white sneakers and canvas bag for an informal afternoon date, jewel sandals and clutch bag for an evening out). On the other hand, **a winter dress** is not only unsuitable for different occasions but also **less versatile—even with regard to the shape of the woman wearing it**—because a pattern that enhances a given body type may not be that flattering on a different one.

It's thus better to go for different garments and pairings based on the season.

In autumn and spring, one of the key pieces for any stylish outfit is undoubtedly a pair of **jeans (or trousers)**. In these seasons you don't have tanned legs and arms to help you look slimmer, nor can you hide leg imperfections under knee-high boots (as you can in the winter). Therefore, **choosing the perfect trousers becomes essential** when picking out your daily ensemble.

If you find a pair of pants (be they jeans or not) that's perfect for your shape, **you can wear it no matter where you need to be**, as it's a baseline garment that never goes out of style. It's versatile enough for your nine-to-five as well as more formal settings.

To look chic and stylish, you don't necessarily need to wear expensive or designer garments: as long as what you're wearing is **in tune with your own inner style and expresses your personality**, a well-made, good-quality, fitted pair of dark jeans paired with a shirt or a top that lights you up may produce an outstanding outcome (and this can be done on a budget).

Always remember that there's nothing less elegant than a woman who doesn't feel comfortable with her clothes (no matter what their price), so **if your style is informal, don't try to wear excessively formal outfits**: a more easygoing choice will make you feel trendy, attractive, and self-confident as no other garment will ever do. **With your perfect jeans, it's up to you to dress them up or down** with the appropriate accessories: flat shoes and a wide bag at work; stiletto heels, costume jewelry, and a smaller bag for a night out.

Here's one more recommendation: when wearing interchangeable baseline garments, **focusing on the details** is essential for a striking look. Hemming your pants to the right length and choosing the right height for your heels can make a difference and transform an ordinary outfit into a chic, trendy, and outstanding one.

These combinations **save time** (and money). They're essential for both superbusy businesswomen and homebodies who want a flawless, easygoing choice for everywhere from the supermarket to the parent-teacher meeting. And they will give you **a simple but sophisticated look**, enhancing your style and your femininity.

11. Straight Jeans

As mentioned before, a foundation piece in spring and autumn is a nice pair of jeans, which—thanks to the countless variations in color, fit, and fabric—can be worn by women of all ages, styles, and body shapes.

As **this item is always trendy**, though, it's sometimes possible to come across one of the thousand designs of the latest trend that may not be suitable for all body types.

The most versatile pattern, which lends itself to different combinations and can be suitable for different figures and styles, is **the ageless straight pattern**, which also has the considerable advantage of being **suitable for pairing with shoes of any kind**. This pattern is classic but always fashionable, and it's **also flattering for curvy figures** (while other patterns aren't).

A straight cut is **also lovely on thin women** who can look excessively skinny with more formfitting styles, and it's also perfect for those who prefer not to wear too-tight cuts.

It's possible to find straight jeans made with **shaping fabrics** or **cuts specifically designed to push up, slim down**, or otherwise make the most of your physical assets.

It's important to point out that if you want to look thinner with this garment, you'd better **focus your attention on the details—** above all the **hem**. As a line that visually breaks the figure, the hem is a **key factor when it comes to enhancing your legs and your whole figure**. If properly hemmed, straight jeans can make you look chic, slim, and sophisticated; but the wrong hem can add unwanted extra pounds while making you look anything but classy.

Here are some tips for a faultless outcome:

(1) **The ideal hem height for straight pants** is usually **at the ankle** (one inch higher than your malleolus if you have thin ankles—slightly lower if your ankle is not very thin). This solution is not only the most versatile but also the most slimming one, as it highlights your ankle—the slimmer part of your leg—and has an overall slimming effect on your figure.

(2) If you hem your straight jeans at the ankle, **you can pair them with any type of shoe**—be they high heels, ballet flats, or sneakers (whereas you can't do the same with longer hems).

As clearly shown in the pictures, when the hem is at the right height (right) **the legs look longer and leaner**, whereas improperly hemmed pants (on the left) enlarge the whole figure.

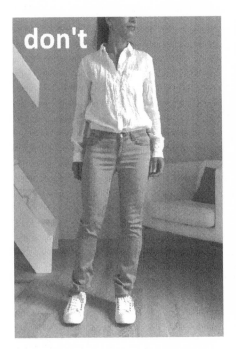 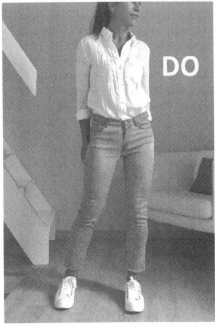

Moreover, if you want a flawless and enhancing result, there are two **things to avoid**:

(1) **Cuffed jeans** (unless the cuff is a tailored one): a cuff visually divides the figure, shortening your legs. And with denim fabrics, it's anything but chic.

(2) **Unhemmed jeans: they wrap themselves around your lower leg** and add unpleasant volume to your ankle and calf.

This rule applies to all body types: even if cuffed (or unhemmed) jeans are in fashion, remember that this doesn't make you chic or slimmer; conversely, they just look dowdy, so it's better to avoid them. **If you want to be chic and classy, it's better to follow your personal style** instead of just following the crowd (especially if the crowd is tasteless).

Cuffed jeans and "ivy" jeans make me think of an old Tuscan saying: "**buy some leg or sell some cloth**," which refers to **pants that are too long for one's legs**. If your intention is to look slimmer and classy, it's better to choose another strategy.

As for color, **the classic medium wash** has the advantage of being neither too bright nor too dark, so it can be **flawlessly paired with many different colors without creating a jarring contrast between your upper and lower body** (which is always helpful for looking slender).

Be careful with excessive acid washing: **if the color is too irregular, it can make your legs look shorter or crooked** due to the fact that the eye perceives clothes (and their variations in color) more than your actual figure. The same goes for fading around the buttocks, which can be useful if you want to look more full figured but is not very helpful if you want to look slimmer in the hips.

The same applies to sidebands, which now are so fashionable. Some think they have a slimming effect, but this is just not the case. In fact, **they make your legs look fuller**, so the outcome is exactly the opposite.

To conclude, here's a practical tip: if you already have jeans with excessive fading, and you realize they are not suitable for your figure, dye them in blue or black instead of getting rid of them; the bright spots will become much less visible, and the enlarging effect will disappear.

12. Flared Jeans

Flared jeans are another wardrobe staple that is totally fashionable, **looks good on everyone**, and has a slimming effect (as long as it's *slightly* flared). The same goes for **boot-cut jeans** (which are tight around the leg and knee but looser at the bottom).

A pair of flared jeans, **when paired with medium-to-high heels, is a must-wear for flattering your silhouette** and getting a taller-looking figure. Since the heel remains hidden, **you can wear shoes with a heel as high as you want** without worrying about any disproportion between heel and legs, thus achieving the pleasant outcome of longer and leaner legs.

Be aware, though, that **too-wide patterns are to be avoided**; otherwise the effect will just be the opposite. Here again it's **essential to hem your flared jeans to the correct height: long enough to cover the heel but no longer**—otherwise it has the unpleasant outcome of widening your leg.

This is the only drawback of this garment. **If you adjust the hem of flared jeans for low-heeled shoes, you can't wear the same pants for high-heeled ones.** (This is unlike straight jeans, which if properly hemmed at the ankle can be worn with any kind of shoes.) A wide trouser that flutters at half length is not only totally tasteless, but it also has a widening effect. Instead of creating an uninterrupted vertical line that slims your silhouette, it just cuts your figure shorter. Similarly, flared jeans with a hem adjusted for high-heeled shoes can't be worn with flat ones, because this would create unpleasant folds that widen the lower leg.

If you always wear heels of the same height, the issue does not even arise, but if you like to alternate shoes, one solution is to **take advantage of a sale and buy two identical jeans** (luckily enough, quality jeans don't need to be expensive), then **adjust the hems to two different heights**. This way, you can take full advantage of this pattern, which can elongate your leg like skinny jeans could never do, as you can see from a comparison between the pictures below.

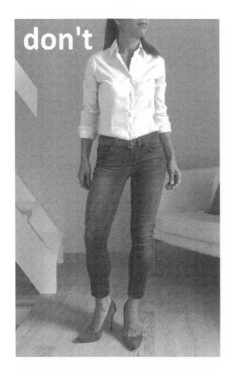 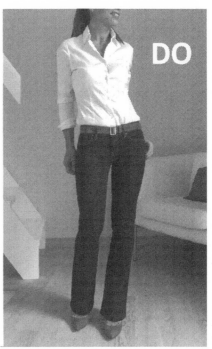

Boot-cut or flared jeans are also **the perfect trousers** to wear **with ankle boots** (conversely, ankle boots may have the drawback of making your legs look shorter when worn with skinny jeans): the boot-cut allows you to hide your ankle boots under the pants, thus **creating a vertical line that stretches your figure out**.

Another point to consider for a flawless outcome concerns the **size and position of back pockets** (this also applies to the straight jeans of the previous chapter). Be aware of the following:

(1) Large, low-back pockets shorten your leg.
(2) Too-small ones could make the buttocks appear fuller.
(3) The same goes for pockets with striking seams, because they can enlarge your figure.

The perfect choice is to opt for **medium-sized pockets** that remain **centered on your buttocks** and have seams that match the color of your trousers. If your butt is not excessively skinny, you can also wear trousers with no back pockets (as long as the pants are well made and properly shaped).

As for combinations, the most flattering solution is to **pair garments whose color is similar** (not necessarily *identical*) to the color of your trousers. A nice alternative to monochrome is the striped shirt mentioned in chapter 2 (as long as the stripes that match the trousers are wide enough to be visible at some distance), and the white shirt.

As for the washes, **excessive bleach or acid washes** are to be avoided because they **may have a widening effect**.

When in doubt, stick with **medium-wash jeans in classic shades (blue, black, and gray)**, which never go out of style. Though this may not coincide with the new trends shown in the stores, this is not your concern: your goal should not be to achieve an up-to-the-minute look (which may become dated in a few months), but a **timeless style** that **will look trendy, stylish, and unique** no matter what the fads say.

13. Black Pants

Another garment that is **suitable to all styles and all body shapes** and can be easily worn with different garments **with a classy and chic outcome** is the black trouser—a garment that if well made and carefully paired, can be **a foundation piece for any occasion**. Even in formal settings or occasions where you do not clearly understand the required dress code, black pants (or black jeans) plus a shirt or a silk top are perfect for a **chic, stylish, and always tasteful look**.

Black pants are neither serious nor boring. They can be made suitable for many occasions simply by changing your accessories. **You can easily dress them up or down depending on where you need to be**, avoiding any risk of looking overdressed or too informal.

This garment has a lot of potential, yet—oddly enough—even if most women wear black trousers, **it's not always easy to choose and match them** in the most appropriate way, so let's see some tips for a faultless choice.

What should certainly be avoided (though something you see very often) is the wide pants in synthetic fabric with a fluttering bottom: it doesn't look good on anyone, and don't believe that a wide bottom makes your hips look thinner, because if it's too wide and not paired with high heels, it will do just the opposite.

The most versatile style is the straight cut, which—similarly to what was previously mentioned about jeans—looks good for most body types, styles, and ages, and lends itself to any possible pairing. The straight pattern, **if properly hemmed at the ankle, can be worn with sneakers as well as stilettos**, thus enhancing its versatility.

A skinny pattern may also be suitable for many as long as it's not a superskinny cut (otherwise it would highlight any imperfections), and it should be paired with garments quite loose for your upper body—avoid any pairing with excessively tight tops.

Conversely, a tight top may be suitable with a boot-cut pattern, because, being broad at the bottom, it balances out the upper part.

As for chromatic combinations, a pair of black trousers **is just perfect with black, white, gray, and with all neutral colors**, whereas pairings with bold-colored tops or sweaters may look quite dated (as well as having a thickening outcome, as you can see in the picture on the left).

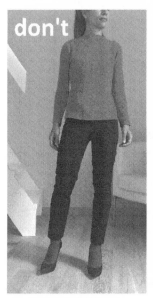 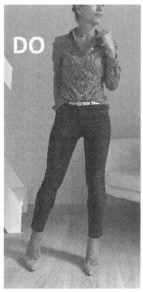 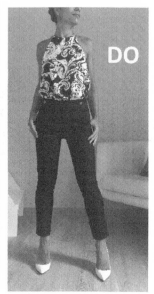

Here are some tips for the perfect choice:

(1) If you think you have a few extra pounds, **avoid trousers that are wide all over your legs: they make things even worse**, because the circumference of your thigh becomes that of your knee and of your ankle. These pants do not hide anything; indeed they do quite the opposite by highlighting what you would like to hide.

(2) Palazzo pants may be an exception to the previous rule, but only if you are very tall and as long as you pair them with heels.

(3) You get the best effect when **the trouser leg falls straight—tight but straight** (it should not wring around your leg).

(4) Belt loops must be thin and close to the trousers, and they should not look like curtain rings.

To look chic and slim, it's better to avoid pockets of any kind. As my coauthor Benedetta always says, "In the most expensive boutiques, where they produce tailor-made trousers to make the most fleshy and aged uptown Milan matrons look lean and elegant, trousers *never* have pockets."

As for fabrics, for a maximum slimming effect, you may choose **well-made shaping fabrics**. If they are of the highest quality, they **will make your legs look more toned, adding a touch of elegance**.

Don't forget a rule that applies to all types of fabric and styles: at the end of the day, **the trousers should not lose their shape around your knees or buttocks**. Pay attention to the material and cut and try to pick out quality items, so you will feel chic and put together throughout the day and not just the first ten minutes.

Remember that when looking for your staple black pants, you must **focus on quality and fit** no matter what the newest trend says: if you feel chic and slim with your straight pants because you have short legs and strong calves, it doesn't matter if the most famous blogger claims the wonder of stretch silk. When it comes to wardrobe staples, just go for what enhances your body and fits your style and taste, regardless of the fads (if they coincide, so much better for you). Trust yourself and **invest your time in searching for the garment that's perfect for you**. In a very short time, your taste will become foolproof, and the results, believe me, will be extraordinary!

14. White Shirt

One of the main staples is undoubtedly the white shirt, which allows you to get **a polished look that's timeless, chic, and even—if you want—extremely sexy** (much more, believe me, than any low-cut sweaters, microtops, or microskirts).

If you find your perfect white shirt, **people will remember you as an attractive, chic, charming, and interesting woman**. They will not say that you were wearing a nice shirt—they will probably not even remember your shirt, but **they will certainly remember** *you*.

A white shirt can make the most of your style, brightening your features and **making you shine** even with a simple, classy look.

On the other hand, since this garment lights up everything around, **its starkness can be a drawback**: it should be avoided if you are not feeling your best, because it highlights imperfections and does not look great with less-than-perfect skin, excessive makeup, untidy hair, and dark circles around the eyes.

Here some tips for an impeccable choice:

(1) Unlike the white T-shirt (which can also be a low-priced garment), **quality is a must** with a white shirt. If you choose a low-quality cut or fabric, all allure goes out the window.

(2) The only exception are loose blouses in synthetic silk: these garments may have lovely results even if their quality is not outstanding.

(3) Stiff fabrics add volume to your figure. It's better to choose fabrics **soft enough to follow your shape without being too tight** or formfitting.

(4) As for colors, stark white produces an outstanding outcome, though in some cases it may be better to soften the tone with off-white or oatmeal instead; these tones are more suitable for certain complexions and may be easier to wear.

(5) If you prefer a **looser pattern**, always **match it with tight-fitted or skinny pants**, because wide garments on both your upper and lower body will make you look fuller.

(6) For informal settings, you can also **layer a wide, boyfriend shirt on a dark monochromatic set** (as in the picture on the left): this solution always has a slimming effect, though the allure of the white shirt, in this case, is slightly reduced.

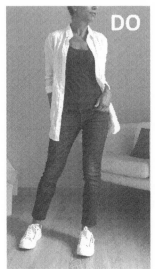 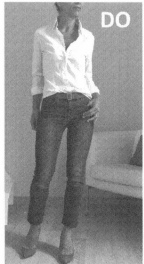 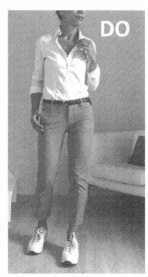

Do not underestimate the details:

- The **buttons** must always be **classic ones**: avoid fanciful buttons; they make the chicest garment lose all its class.
- **Avoid ruffly shirts**; not only is it difficult to find quality items, but they can also **make you look more full-bodied**. A ruffle-sleeve shirt stretches out your arms and by contrast makes your legs look shorter (not to mention it makes you look like a flamenco dancer).
- Conversely, if you wear your white shirt with the **sleeves rolled up**, this visually reduces the length of your arms, **making your legs look comparatively longer**.
- **Rhinestones and sequins are inadmissible on a white shirt**—they are the opposite of elegance. More acceptable are pearls (which can also be used for buttons).

It's also better to **avoid shirts that clearly show their brand**. You don't need any signature with your perfect white shirt—just *yours*: the one that comes from your inner style and unique personality.

Still on the subject of fabrics, the synthetic percentage, if higher than zero (synthetic materials can be useful for a better fit), must be quite low. The fabric should be soft, and the yarn should remain the same over time. For cotton garments, **the higher the cotton quality, the easier it is to iron**.

Shirts made of **opaque silk (be it natural or synthetic)** are good for everyone and **can be worn in many different settings** with jeans and sneakers, with your sexiest stilettos, or with a tailored blazer. These shirts are chameleonic—you can wear them with your favorite medium-wash jeans at twenty, with black trousers and pumps at thirty or forty, with a classic tweed suit (Chanel style) at sixty and older.

A white shirt with these characteristics is a fundamental garment for any woman. **You can easily dress it up or down depending on where you need to be**, and you'll never look too informal or too elegant because **your white shirt will always match perfectly with the rest of your look.** Just change your shoes, and you'll be ready for anything from a business meeting to happy hour.

An easy combination is straight pants (or fitted jeans) and flats for informal settings, but if you remove the flats and add a pair of heels, you are ready for a night out.

If you need to walk, you can also pair this outfit with nice light-colored sneakers and a beautiful bag for **a timeless ensemble** that, beyond being comfortable and classy, will instantly enhance your allure.

15. Lightweight Knit Sweater

Sweaters and jerseys are two of the average woman's most frequent new purchases. It seems like we never get enough of them—not just because every season we find new appealing colors on display in stores but also because **they seemingly don't require any particular attention in the choice,** and therefore the purchase is easier. Hands up if you ever bought a cute $19.99 knit without thinking twice and then only wore it for the first ten days.

In this chapter, we will see some tips on how to choose your perfect lightweight fine-knit sweater—one that **enhances your figure while working with everything** from your signature straight jeans to classic trousers.

A garment like this will stay in your wardrobe for years and still remain trendy and fashionable: for this reason, you'd better **focus on the quality** (instead of quantity) **and look for the perfect fit.**

When chasing your perfect knit, you should **forget about trendy, bold-colored items.** When producing garments with the latest color trends, manufacturers do not invest in quality for items that are not supposed to be worn beyond the first few months (if ever).

Beyond that, since the sweater is right next to your face, choosing bright colors may not be the perfect option for your complexion.

Also, **contrasting colors shorten your figure and are not that chic** (as you will see below in the picture on the left).

As for patterns, avoiding fancy ones is a must when it comes to picking out your foundation pieces.

It's better to go for sweaters in **neutral tones** (be they blue, gray, black, camel, or buttermilk, depending on your complexion) **and minimal styles.**

The quality of yarn must be high—your knit must never lose its shape nor be susceptible to pilling, forcing you to buy an identical one year after year. Instead, you can start exploring a range of colors that may suit you more.

Don't forget that your knit sweater must not follow fashion but your shape and style. It's no coincidence that knits made of quality materials such as cashmere always have classic designs, whereas seasonal garments are always made from less precious fabrics.

The most versatile cuts are **V-neck** (low cut or not), **boatneck, and crew neck**, and the trendier among us should remember that **there are still infinite options**: tight, soft, long (for pairings with skinny pants), or short (for classic or high-waisted trousers). The same goes for colors: neutral shades are endlessly fashionable, and create an outcome that is so much more interesting than some questionable hue that, in addition to not being the most flattering for your complexion, also enlarges the figure, as you will see in the picture on the left.

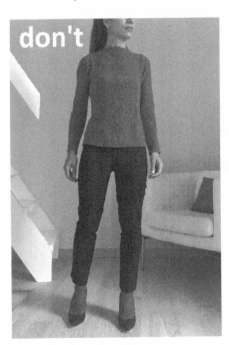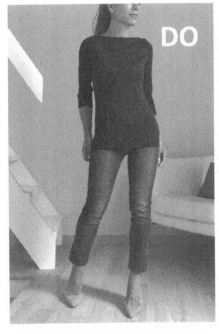

Here some suggestions to help you identify the most suitable design for you:

(1) If you would like to look **thinner**, a **low neckline** is essential, because it always makes your figure look slimmer.

(2) Very wide sweaters do not always help camouflage extra pounds: it may be better to go for a straight cardigan worn open with a darker top and trousers, which always makes your whole figure look thinner.

(3) **Crew-neck patterns enlarge your neck**, widening your bust: if you want to look slimmer, **a boatneck can be the perfect option—being wide, it makes the neck look longer and more slender by contrast** (as seen above in the picture on the right).

(4) **Wide shoulders** are not the most appropriate choice if you are short-statured (like I am), because they **enlarge your whole figure**, creating a thick line that shortens your body.

With your perfect knit, you will get **maximum versatility from morning to night**. A lightweight, dark sweater made of a quality fabric paired with dark skinny or straight trousers, nice shoes, and a nice scarf (or costume jewelry) will work everywhere (for a party, just wear a nice sleeveless silk top under your sweater).

Cashmere used to be considered the most luxurious material, but nowadays that's not always the case. Due to the appeal of this undeniably soft fabric, **many brands are producing cashmere garments that do not last beyond the first washing**, not to mention all that pilling (a little pilling is normal for cashmere due to the fact that its hair is shorter than, for instance, merino). Unless you're totally sure of the quality of the yarn, **it may be better to buy an excellent merino sweater**—one that doesn't pill and doesn't lose its shape even after endless washings—**than a low-quality cashmere sweater**. Among other things, cashmere always requires some attention (brushing, washing, and ironing it the right way). If you are always in a rush, go for lambswool, merino, or mixed wool-silk blends, which are easier to deal with.

Also, note that **the quality does not necessarily match the price**: speaking from personal experience, I have noticed that **some inexpensive brands sell better garments than more exclusive ones**. It's up to you to find the brand that suits you best: have fun with it, and you'll discover less-known quality brands that sell excellent garments!

And **if you ever plan a trip to Italy**, don't forget to find time to **browse a neighborhood market**, where sometimes it's possible to pick out **top-quality inventory garments for just a few Euros**. To be certain that they really come from inventories—unsold clothing bought by weight in bulk and therefore sold at a price even lower than their value—be sure that they come in colors and patterns completely different from one another (otherwise they not real inventory garments but just low-quality, low-priced garments!).

16. Short Jacket

A short jacket is a garment that, though considered a wardrobe staple, isn't really, or at least not always, due to the fact that it isn't suitable for all body types. This is particularly true when talking about the so-called **biker jacket** which, having **broad shoulders** and being **double-breasted**, is **not that flattering if you want to look chic and thinner** and is only suitable for just a few body shapes. Broad shoulders can help camouflage extra volume around the hips only for those who have a huge disproportion (for instance, if you are a size 2 in the shoulders while wearing a size 8 for your hips), but in other cases it's just the opposite, as adding volume in the shoulder area makes the whole figure look fuller.

Conversely, short jackets that have a basic pattern and are *not* double breasted can **indeed be very trendy and stylish** as well as suitable for different body types.

To wear this item faultlessly, though, it's essential to pay attention to the proportions of your body and the garments you wear.

Generally speaking, the easiest solution is to layer a slightly longer garment (be it a knit sweater, a shirt, or a top) under the short jacket and pair it with **skinny or tapered pants**.

The jacket should **preferably be worn open** in order to lengthen your silhouette (as in the photo on the right); when it's too cold to leave it open, you can add a scarf (see chapter 29 for details).

Also, a short jacket is **the perfect option when wearing wide trousers**. With high-waisted wide trousers, a short jacket is a must if you do not want to look like your grandmother; this outfit highlights your waist and helps camouflage any extra pounds around your hips and thighs, giving you a youthful and entrancing look. Similarly, a short jacket **can be faultlessly matched with very long, ample skirts**, white sneakers, and a white T-shirt.

Be aware, however, that for a faultless and chic outcome, the short jacket must be **lightweight**, as padded short jackets may enlarge your figure.

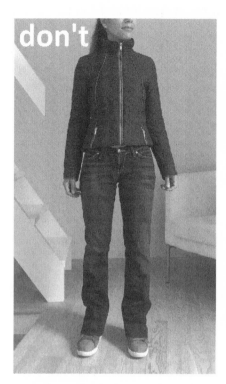 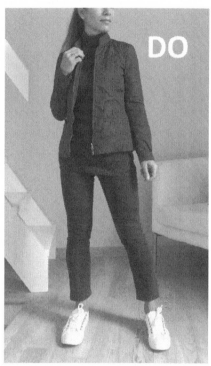

Turning now to the famous **Chanel jacket**—this is certainly a stunning piece, though it **doesn't look good on everyone**. Having a slightly squared shape, if combined with a knee-skirt, it widens your hips cutting your figure shorter (you can achieve a better result by **pairing it with trousers, as long as they are quite tapered**).

Shoes are another important element to consider when wearing a short jacket: unless pairing with palazzo pants (which always require high heels hidden under the trousers), **the perfect shoe option for a short jacket is flat shoes** (as well as sneakers). This is because a short jacket is a visual breakpoint, so adding any other breakpoint (like a heel in plain sight) should be avoided.

Things may be different, though, if you pick out a **jacket** that is **slightly longer**, which—though being less common than the classic pattern—can be easily paired with many garments and is suitable for many body types. The ideal pattern should **cover the**

buttocks and have a belt. This style is particularly suitable for those who would like to look taller; since it hides the upper part of your leg, it camouflages its real length (conversely, a jacket that comes to the waistline can't make your legs look longer).

One last detail: if you choose an item with a **zipper of a different color** from the fabric, this may have a **widening effect**, as you can see in the picture on the left. Like pants with sidebands mentioned in chapter 11, a zipper of a different color becomes a breakpoint that enlarges your figure.

If you already have such a garment, an easy solution is to **match it with a scarf in a color similar to that of the trousers**. This simple trick, in addition to having a **flattering effect**, can also elevate your look, as a low-quality zipper is frequently the only clue that the jacket you're wearing is a cheap one; if you strategically hide it with a well-chosen scarf, it will slim your silhouette **and make your whole outfit look more chic and sophisticated**: win-win!

17. Trench Coat

When talking about outerwear, one of the foundation pieces is the classic trench coat, which beyond being a timeless garment that never goes out of style, **can look good on everyone** and **works with everything** from jeans and sneakers to a dress with heels.

This garment can be worn by every woman, regardless of her age and style, and it's stylish even when it's not the latest trend, because **it's always chic yet informal and practical**.

Its combinations are almost endless; it lends itself to countless pairings with both casual and elegant outfits, allowing you to fine-tune the character of your look to where you need to be.

Since it's tight around the waist (without being too close-fitting) and wide at the bottom, it can enhance your figure, visually extending your silhouette and **shaping and highlighting your curves instead of covering them**. This allows you to camouflage a few extra pounds around the hips, thighs, and also, in part, around the waistline.

A trench is not only suitable for spring and autumn: you can find coats made with **heavier fabrics that are totally suitable for winter** as well as lightweight ones that can be worn in summer showers (they are so lightweight that you can nonchalantly fold and stash them into your bag as soon as the sun comes back).

In addition, a trench is a garment that, despite having a well-defined character, can **emphasize your personal style**. If made well and in a quality fabric, it can make the inexpensive dress you wear underneath seem like a designer one.

Another perk of the trench coat is that its shape, which is wider at the knee, may **visually reduce your buttocks while at the same time slimming your lower leg**. Its belt helps to slim your silhouette, as you can see from the comparison between the photos below (and if you tie the belt slightly above your waist as I did, this can make your legs look longer).

As for color, **neutral hues are the most versatile**. Traditional beige can be found in warmer shades and colder ones; you can always find the tone that best suits your complexion (or otherwise you can add a darker scarf, as in the picture on the right).

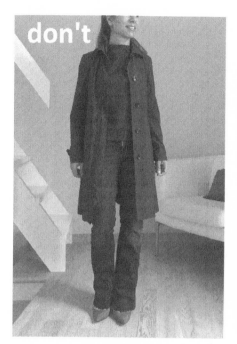
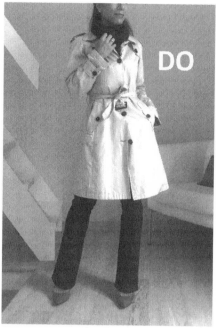

If you are of medium height, the classic design that comes to the knee and is worn tightly at the waist is perfect for you. **If you're short-statured**, it's better to **choose a design that ends above the knee**, because it helps your legs look longer.

For those with a curvy figure, the perfect option is a trapezium shape—preferably paired with tapered trousers.

There are also longer designs, but only the really tall should wear them. The flared style that ends under the knee is stylish and very chic, but if you are not tall, it must be paired with high heels.

As for the choice of trousers, wide ones must be avoided, better to go for **boot-cut quite tight on the knee, or straight pants**.

Be aware that when wearing a trench coat, **your lower leg must be impeccable**, so avoid shapeless pants, random hems, and lengths that are not suitable for you.

Pay attention to the color of your trousers: if you **pair a light-colored trench with dark trousers**, the outcome will be perfect, while the opposite won't; a dark trench layered over light-colored trousers widens your legs, cutting your figure shorter. For this reason, this pairing is suitable only for those who have long, lean legs. For others, a dark trench coat should always be paired with dark trousers.

One more thing to consider: since the trench coat is a very trendy garment, you may also find in stores fancy prints or bright colors that do not have the versatility of a classic design. For this reason, it's essential to pay some attention when shopping for a trench coat. **Before buying a flashy design or color** (which can be fun if well chosen but still has limited versatility), **you must have your perfect staple trench in your closet**.

Also, don't forget that now you can also find lovely overcoats that, even if they are made with different fabrics (wool, for instance), still have a pattern similar to that of the classic trench. These garments may offer a smart and elegant way **to take advantage this style**—which, as explained, looks good on many—**even with different materials**: an extra tool to elevate your look and enhance your chic style.

18. Light-Colored Sneakers

Sneakers are one of the most recent wardrobe staples: for decades mainly worn by younger girls, **they gradually became a real foundation piece for women of all ages**—an item suitable not only for informal settings but also for occasions where formal shoes used to be a must. And this is a good thing, as it means that nowadays sneakers **can even be worn with formal outfits**, allowing incomparable comfort.

A well-chosen sneaker can be paired with even the simplest ensemble of a white shirt and straight jeans with excellent results: **add a nice belt and a quality bag**, and you have an outfit that is **pleasantly casual, stylish, and trendy**.

Many businesswomen in the city also match sneakers with a pantsuit, thus getting a faultless and practical outcome.

A pair of sneakers may also be **worn with a straight knee-length skirt**: this outfit, which used to be worn only by young girls, is now also worn by the most elegant ladies with a very nice effect.

To achieve an impeccable look, however, choose carefully: in stores, you can find any pattern you want in countless styles and colors. Instead of simplifying the choice, this makes your purchase quite difficult.

As this type of shoe is by its very nature a sporty one, **it should preferably be light-colored or bright-colored**, whereas the **darker colors (black above all) are not the most appropriate**. Why? First of all, because choosing a dark color (traditionally reserved for more formal garments) for an informal shoe may seem like an attempt to formalize an item that doesn't—and shouldn't—have any formal character. The **allure of sneakers lies in their breezy look**, and any attempt to cover them with a formal coating will take their appeal away.

Secondly, **light-colored sneakers visually elongate your legs (and your whole figure)**, while dark ones simply *don't*.

Since sneakers entirely cover your foot and have no heel, it's essential to opt for light neutral tones (or at least moderately bright ones) if you want to have some kind of slimming effect.

Light-colored sneakers may elongate your figure, **making your legs look thinner**, as you can see in the comparison between the photos below.

The dark sneakers on the left, despite having a two-inch wedge, cut the figure shorter, whereas the white ones enhance the silhouette, making it look more proportional.

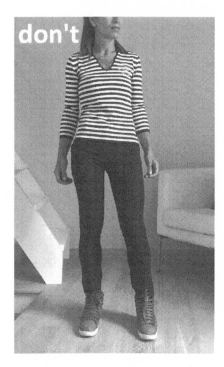 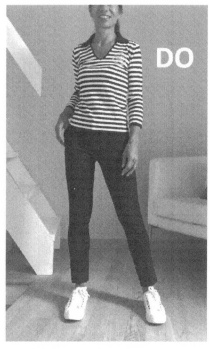

Speaking of light colors, we don't necessarily mean white: **beige, light gray, buttermilk, taupe**, and many other neutral shades can work as well. As an alternative to light colors, you may also use some **intense hues as long as they are not too dark**.

To elongate your bottom half and flatter your silhouette, **pair your sneakers with straight or tapered pants hemmed at the ankle** (as mentioned earlier when talking about straight pants) and *don't* wear socks (or opt for invisible ones. Fishnet socks may be another interesting and very sexy option) in order to highlight the slimmer part of your leg, thus making you look thinner and taller.

This trick, by the way, **also works if you don't have very thin ankles**, because **in any case, they would look considerably thinner than they are** (and in addition the outcome will be very chic and fashionable).

As for the heel, **the ideal sneaker should have no wedge** or at least a very low one (as long as it's imperceptible).

If you don't have thin legs, avoid high sneakers (which cover the ankle), because they may cut your figure shorter. If you are not very tall but love high sneakers, you can wear them with dark, straight pants in the same color as the shoe (this is the only case where dark-colored sneakers may flatter your figure) or pair them with boot-cut or flared trousers that hide the shoe.

Avoid platforms at all costs: not only they do *not* have any slimming effect, but they also take class away from your look, **they don't make you look taller, and they don't make your legs longer** but just give the impression that you're standing right above an imaginary step with your short legs. It's better to forget it, don't you agree?

19. Pumps

Pumps, interestingly enough, have a story that goes exactly in the opposite direction than that of the sneakers.

A fundamental article for every woman a few decades ago, today they are no longer an everyday, every-woman item. This is too bad, because **nice pumps can add femininity and class to your look**, and **they may also be perfectly comfortable**.

With a well-made shoe, you can feel as elegant as an actress on the red carpet even if you wear inexpensive jeans and a plain white tee. On the other hand, **when wearing ugly shoes—or shoes not suitable for you—you can look frumpy** (rather than chic and sophisticated) **even if you wear designer clothes.**

In this chapter, we will see some tips to help you **pick out the perfect shoes for your body type**—shoes that can help you stretch your silhouette and get a chic, timeless look and can be worn in any setting with outstanding results.

Be aware that a quality shoe with the pattern most appropriate for your body shape **can turn an ordinary outfit into a trendy and fashionable look**; it's a good thing to take advantage of this fact!

Those who don't habitually wear high-heeled shoes should know that a two-inch heel, if it's well made, will not only make you appear more feminine but may also be worn with total ease all day long—as long as you **choose a comfortable leather shoe in a design that's easy to wear**.

Here are some tips for a faultless choice:

(1) Avoid not only too-tight models but also too large ones: apart from the Cinderella effect, a shoe that slips away from your feet can be as uncomfortable as a shoe that is too tight.

(2) **The softness of the material is essential** for perfect comfort. Unfortunately, some expensive brands use a very stiff leather, so be careful in your purchases, and don't forget that **your walk should be feminine and sensual**. If your feet are covered with blisters, your walk will seem that of a drunk marathon runner—certainly not that of a catwalk diva.

(3) Choose heels that **complement the shape of your legs**: **for curvy figures**, for example, wide heels and slightly rounded toes help a lot, whereas **excessively pointy toes and thin heels** should be avoided, because they can **create an unflattering disproportion**.

(4) Similarly, **the height of the heel should be proportional to the length of your lower leg**. If you are not very tall, remember that—even if you crave very high heels—you should always look for a proportional shoe. **A heel that's too high will make your legs look shorter by contrast**, so if you want a harmonious and chic effect, it's smarter to wear a lower heel. It's also smart to choose shoes that are similar to your skin tone instead of higher heels in a contrasting color, which can shorten your figure. Otherwise, wear trousers that cover the whole heel.

Shorter women should also avoid straight heels. The perfect option is a slightly curved heel placed centrally under the heel of your foot: this trick, in addition to making the shoe more comfortable when walking, visually reduces the heel's height, and the outcome is therefore more proportioned.

For a slimming effect, **a minimal design is preferable**, as it leaves your feet as visible as possible. The more skin you show, the more your legs are visually stretched out.

Platform pumps should not even be taken into consideration—no matter what the trends say. As my coauthor Benedetta says, "If you are not Gisele or Gigi Hadidi, they concentrate all the weight toward your lower part, like the clogs of a cow." Forget it.

When buying your perfect heels, remember that (1) this type of shoe **must be high quality** and (2) **quality does not necessarily mean expensive**: a well-made shoe from a not-so-expensive brand can be worth much more than the designer shoe that's inappropriate for your body type.

Avoid brands that change designs every year: manufacturers that know how to make great shoes never change their staple models. Top brands generally have a "staple" production of

perfect, timeless, and never-changing designs (why change perfection?). These items may be very expensive, so **study their design and look for similar but more affordable ones elsewhere**.

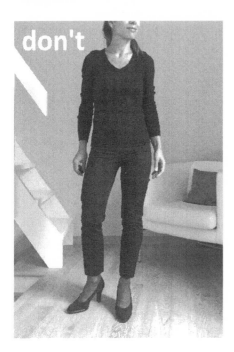
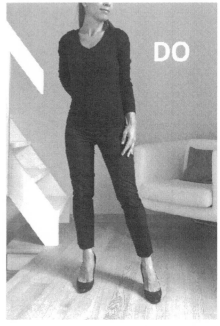

If you want to treat yourself with a pair of heels from your favorite designer, don't forget that **you can find a great deal on outstanding shoes if you are patient and keep looking** (online shops may help). The colors you end up with may not be the most neutral, but don't forget that **bright-colored heels can liven up a dark, monochromatic outfit**.

Speaking from personal experience, since I usually wear neutral hues for my clothes, I intentionally choose bright or intense hues for my pumps (preferably the warmer tones for an extra slimming effect, like yellow, orange, and red, or deeper ones like burgundy). I use them **to lighten up an all-gray, all-black, or all-blue outfit**, thus creating a trendy and stylish ensemble.

One last detail: after the purchase, don't forget to maintain your heels. They must *always* be **shiny and clean**. One trick to clean them easily and quickly is to **use baby wipes** (they're not just for diapers!), which have delicate yet powerful cleansing agents. Never wear the same pair two days straight: **shoes must have time to fully dry before you wear them again**; otherwise they will look old and lose their shape in a few weeks.

These small details will help you wear your perfect pumps impeccably, providing you with **an extra tool to achieve a stylish, timeless, and chic look.**

20. Lightweight Scarf

A lightweight scarf, though seemingly unnecessary, can indeed **help make your figure more proportional**, as it visually reduces the length of your bust, making your legs longer by contrast. For this reason, scarves and pashminas are **real foundation pieces for a stylish look**. They look good on every woman regardless of her age and body shape. If smartly chosen and paired, they can **add class to your outfit** and make you feel **chic and polished even with the most informal garments**. In addition, they can give the appearance of a leaner figure.

Throwing a silk scarf around your neck can make even a simple T-shirt look sophisticated, and a scarf can have **stunning results with the simplest jeans, elevating your look** in seconds.

Slightly different from the classic silk scarf, a **pashmina scarf**—not only the classic cashmere one but ones made of a variety of fabrics—is another item that may be particularly suitable for spring and summer thanks to the fact that it **allows you to adjust your look to suit any weather**. You may also wear it on your shoulders in cooler summer evenings and use it as a **practical yet stylish garment to enhance your style**.

The main difference between a silk scarf and a pashmina scarf is that the second can be used as a real garment—as an alternative to a jacket, for instance—whereas a silk scarf usually cannot.

Furthermore, a silk scarf, though being perfect in spring and autumn, is not very suitable for summer and winter, whereas a pashmina scarf can also be worn as a stole in summer or layered with a coat in winter.

As for the pairings, there are two different ways of taking advantage of these versatile pieces:

(1) A **scarf with an intense tone** may be used to **add a dash of color to an ensemble of dark tones**.
(2) A **scarf in a neutral hue** (gray, blue, taupe) may be **layered over a bright-colored coat or jacket**, thus diminishing the impact of bold colors on your complexion.

Stashing a scarf in your handbag will allow you to quickly adjust your outfit to temperature changes with elegance and nonchalance—similar to what a linen shirt can do in summer.

With regard to the purchase, it's usually possible to buy designer scarves on sale at a reasonable cost and find fine-looking items and beautiful colors and prints at inexpensive prices, though the choice may not be that easy. **Geometric patterns are ageless**—as are fancy patterns with asymmetrical prints and colors. The **classic equestrian style, if it's *your* style, is a fine choice**, and it's always pleasant. If you often dress in neutral colors like black, white, and gray, a **black-and-white print** is a gorgeous and versatile choice that can boost your look in an instant.

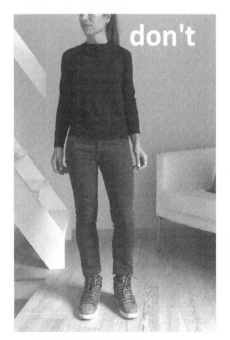 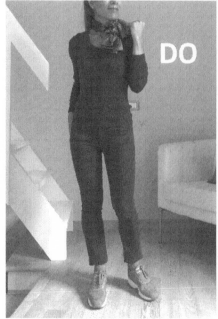

Conversely, **I would not recommend big floral prints to anyone** for many reasons. First of all, scarves in mediocre floral prints are constantly present in many low-quality department stores and can make your outfit appear a bit confused. Also, floral patterns are frequently intended to be worn by fragile and delicate women. **If you're anything but fragile** and your only delicate part is the tip of your nose, then **it's better to opt for patterns more in tune with your character**. The results will surely be better.

For lightweight scarves it's better to give preference to **shiny textiles (silk above all**, be it natural or synthetic), as they brighten your face; conversely, **opaque fabrics are usually easier to pair when talking about pashminas**.

Don't forget that a lightweight scarf may also be used in many other different ways:

(1) You may **use it as a belt**.
(2) You can **tie it to the handles of your handbag** (this adds a touch of class, and it's helpful to protect the handles, which can be easily damaged).
(3) With a few knots, you can also turn it into a stylish shopping bag!

An extra tip: scarves, pashminas, and stoles are **the ideal purchase when you go abroad**. In different countries you can find **stunning, handcrafted products** in a variety of patterns, textures, colors, and fabrics. Keep this in mind for your next trip, and you will bring home a souvenir that you won't forget in a drawer—one that will enhance your look in a totally chic and timeless way.

PART 3

10 Wardrobe Essentials for Winter Clothing

Wardrobe Essentials for Winter Clothing

When it comes to winter clothing, it's important to keep in mind that the **quality of the fabric** becomes **an essential element**. In the summer choosing a 100 percent linen garment is a chic and always classy choice, and in spring your perfect-fit jeans are a versatile and timeless option, but in winter the choice may not be that easy: to play it safe, it's essential to stick to quality pieces.

There are various reasons why quality is so important in the winter months. First, winter fabrics are heavier, which makes a poor-quality fabric immediately visible, and this cannot be camouflaged in any way. Even the cuts take on a greater importance. **When layering many garments, it is essential to choose well-made ones**—otherwise you'll look all bundled up. A garment made of a beautiful fabric and cleverly sewn can **enhance your style and make the most of your physical assets**, while the same garment but awkwardly sewn and in a poor-quality fabric can add unpleasant extra pounds (and bulk) to your figure.

When it's cold, the clothes are closer to your face, and there is no filter provided (like bare arms in the summer or low necklines in spring), so the quality of the garment should be outstanding. **A lovely fabric may brighten your face and flatter your silhouette**, whereas a poor-quality one can make you look frumpy and dowdy, enlarging your figure.

That said, it is also true that identifying the most flattering fabrics, textures, and cuts is not always that easy, given that you may find quality items from cheaper brands, and an expensive garment may not always produce a faultless outcome.

For this reason, it's always essential to **take your time** when making your choices.
Buy less but wisely.
Invest your time in researching the item that is just perfect for you instead of buying your twentieth cheap black acrylic sweater.

Maybe this will require some time, but you will see that your efforts will shortly be rewarded!

21. Turtleneck Sweater

In the cold season, turtleneck sweaters are very versatile: these garments can be considered a real staple because they lend themselves to different styles, are **appropriate for many settings**, and can create different looks depending on how you pair them. A turtleneck bypasses any doubt that may arise when pairing a shirt with a knit, and it also **flatters your silhouette in an easy and comfortable way**.

This garment can give you **an elegant and sophisticated look** and—surprisingly enough—can be incredibly helpful for anyone with a short neck. A well-made turtleneck can perfectly camouflage a short neck, which is conversely highlighted by a crew-neck sweater.

The truth is that the turtleneck can **make your neck seem longer, thus lengthening your whole silhouette**, whereas a crew-neck highlights a short neck and makes it look larger, producing an overall widening effect, as you will see in the comparison between the two pictures below.

Finding the design that's most suitable to your body shape is quite simple. Here are some tips to identify the one that suits you best:

(1) If you have **a few extra pounds around your waistline** and proportionally thinner legs, the ideal pattern is **a broad one** that covers the buttocks. This can be **paired with skinny pants that will slim the figure**.

(2) If you have **a thin waistline but bigger hips and legs**, the perfect choice is a **close-fitting turtleneck** with a tight-fitting collar. **Pair this with a flared skirt** that's narrow at the waist and looser at the bottom: it will highlight your waist, and your hips will go unnoticed.

(3) A wide breast is highlighted by a tight-fitting turtleneck much more than a tight-fitting crew neck, so if you like to emphasize your curves, this is just perfect. For those who feel more comfortable when their breast is not highlighted, it's better to choose slightly looser patterns.

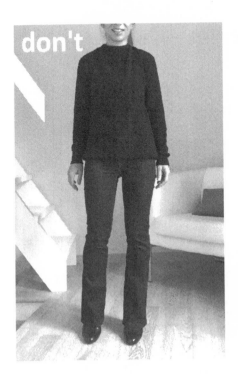
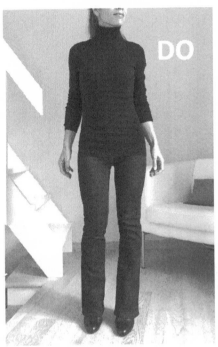

In my opinion, **only those who think they are overweight all over should avoid turtlenecks**: it may be better for these women to **opt for a low-neckline sweater in a dark color that matches the pants**. This always has a slimming effect and enhances your physical assets while hiding what you want to hide. The turtleneck, despite being a garment that generally helps slim the silhouette, is suitable for those who have slimmer body parts to highlight (even if it's just your wrists), because **it emphasizes the thinner parts of the figure**. But if you are decidedly curvy all over, a low neckline may be more helpful to make your figure appear slimmer.

In any case, always **avoid wearing a turtleneck under another sweater**: except for the classic twinset, such combinations are seldom successful and can make you look like a hiker ready for an expedition in the Himalayas. It's better to opt for a very heavy turtleneck *under* which you may put all the sweaters you want—but do not add anything *above* the turtleneck.

Remember that **you should only wear plain and simple garments under a turtleneck**; the perfect option is a close-fitting sweater (be it sleeveless or short sleeved), whereas wearing a shirt under a turtleneck may have a bundling effect.

A slim-fitting turtleneck may also be worn under a blazer: this ensemble is perfect even at work, and if you pair a **dark turtleneck and dark trousers with a bright-colored coat** (or jacket), you'll get a very trendy and stylish look.

This is indeed an extremely versatile garment that can look good on anyone in any setting: **with black trousers, heels, and a beautiful necklace, it's perfect for an evening out**, while the same turtleneck paired with dark jeans and sneakers becomes very suitable even for informal occasions.

Be aware, though, that when talking about staples, **we only mean solid-color turtlenecks**: fancy ones are all but versatile and very seldom chic (striped ones may be an exception but not always). For this ageless piece, it's better to stay on the safe side, and if you want to spice up your look, you can choose some unusual knit.

The same goes for colors: as the turtleneck is close to your face (there is no visual filter provided by the neckline), it's better to **stick with neutral shades and avoid bright ones**, only choosing colors that work best for your skin tone.

And if the whole ensemble seems too dark, you can always **light it up with a striking necklace**, which among other things—as we will see later in chapter 27—is another key accessory that always helps you look thinner, polished, and chic.

22. Skinny Jeans

Skinny jeans, which in other seasons may not be easy to wear, in winter become a very versatile staple that can be worn on a daily basis. They **allow you to balance any extra volume in your upper body**—which in cooler months is quite common—thanks to a minimal design that helps harmonize the silhouette.

It's usually quite easy to pick out the item most suitable for you: a pair of skinny jeans **can be bought at an inexpensive price**, so you can get faultless results even with cheaper brands (though you should choose carefully to get a nice fit and good wearability).

The first thing to say is that the fabric should be stretchy, though **the elasticity of the material**—which depends on the percentage of elastane—**should not be excessive**. If the amount of elastane is about 3–4 percent, the wearability is just perfect, and the shaping effect is maximum. If it's lower (1–2 percent), the jeans could end up being quite uncomfortable (unless it contains a little percentage of polyester or other synthetic fibers). Percentages over 4 or 5 percent should generally be avoided, because the fabric can lose its shaping effect, and the jeans become excessively loose fitting in a few hours.

When it comes to choosing a size, don't forget that **with jeans, when in doubt, it's better to opt for smaller** to avoid an involuntary baggy effect on your buttocks or around your hips (which would not be chic or feminine) caused by the stretch fabric becoming a little looser over time.

As for colors—as previously mentioned in the chapters on straight and boot-cut jeans—**excessively faded jeans** or acid washings with stark contrasts **may highlight imperfections and enlarge your figure**. The same goes for light-blue or light-colored jeans. **If you like light-colored jeans, it's safer to pick out a white pair** as long as it has a nice cut and is made of a quality fabric. Well-made white jeans don't have the widening effect that excessively washed-out jeans may have.

The most versatile color—the one that you can faultlessly match with any other tonality—**is the classic medium-dark**

blue, but **you may also have impeccable results with black, gray, and all dark shades**.

Be wary of bold colors, as they can easily show their low quality (and moreover, if you wear bold-colored jeans with a medium-length coat, this could make your legs look shorter).

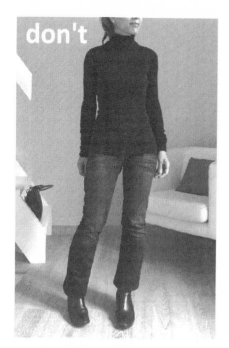 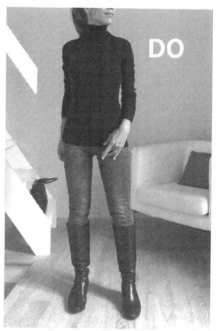

Regarding pairings, here some suggestions:

(1) To impeccably wear *super*skinny jeans, you should have perfectly proportional, tapered legs (not too skinny). An easier option, which usually looks good on everyone, is to **opt for skinny jeans that are slightly wider from the knee down instead of superskinny ones**; if the fabric is extra-tight around the ankle, it may highlight imperfections while making your legs look shorter. For this reason medium-skinny styles are usually preferable to ultraskinny ones, which look good only on those who have long and perfectly tapered legs.

(2) **Skinny jeans are perfect when paired with knee-high boots**, as long as your upper leg (thighs and hips) is

proportional (which does *not* necessarily mean thin); conversely, if you wore straight or boot-cut jeans over knee-high boots, this would give the appearance of a bulkier and shorter leg (as you can see from the comparison between the pictures above).

(3) For those who want to **camouflage a few extra pounds around the hips**, it's better to pair skinny jeans with a wide knit sweater that covers the buttocks and with **ankle boots in the same color of the jeans**; the ankle boots should preferably be quite tight around the ankle so as to stretch the legs, visually creating a long, vertical line.

(4) **Avoid any combination of skinny jeans and low-heeled ankle boots that are loose around the ankle**: this pairing is only suitable for teenagers or those who have very thin legs, because it shortens your legs—and your whole figure— making you look seem fuller (and besides, it's anything but chic).

Skinny jeans may not be a suitable option only **for those who have a strong calf *and* not-so-long legs**. Regardless of your weight and height, in this case **it's better to opt for boot-cut styles worn with high-heeled ankle boots** as long as the heel remains hidden under the flare (which always lengthens and slims the leg and the whole figure).

As for the many styles on display in store windows, be aware that skinny jeans with **irregular fading** (which now are totally fashionable) **can make even perfectly straight legs look crooked** due to the fact that the eye perceives the clothes you're wearing much more than your actual shape. So if you choose trousers with stark contrasts in their color, this could visually change the shape of your legs.

23. Knit Dress

The dress, a real statement piece in the summer, is not so easy to wear flawlessly in the cooler months. This is mainly due to the fact that **the versatility of a summer dress comes not only from its light fabric** (which gently follows your figure without enlarging it) **but also from the fact that it's usually sleeveless**, creating an uninterrupted vertical line that gives the impression of a slimmer (and more elegant) figure.

In the winter months, though, things are completely different. The patterns are not so flattering (**a flared dress made with a heavy fabric has a decidedly worse wearability** than its lightweight sister, and it can easily bunch up, making you look bulky instead of feminine and graceful). Also, the **sleeves add extra volume to your upper body**, visually doubling its size and **enlarging your whole figure** (this does not happen when wearing a trousers-sweater combination, because pants allow the shape of your legs to be seen).

Furthermore, wearing a dress in winter is a not-so-versatile option, as **a winter dress has its own well-defined character**: the same dress can hardly be suitable for any setting.

An interesting option for feminine ladies who love this garment is to wear a sleeveless sheath dress over a dark, slim-fitting sweater and pairing this outfit with dark, opaque stockings and dark shoes: with this ensemble the dress keeps its simple and straight line, producing a nice outcome—though this outfit doesn't look good on everyone (as you can see below in the picture on the left).

A more versatile alternative may be a knit dress (picture on the right). Though this garment is by nature quite casual and easygoing, it can achieve **a lovely balance between looking informal and polished** in the cooler months, and it's also suitable for many different body types.

This item, when paired with dark, opaque stockings and dark knee-high boots, can **flatter your figure so much more than**

many formal dresses, and if you add some good-quality accessories, you can easily dress it up or down depending on where you need to be.

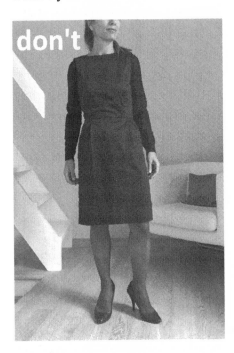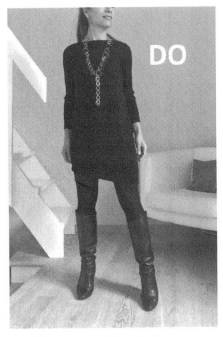

Here are some suggestions for a faultless outcome:

(1) **A knit dress must always be single colored.** Whatever your weight and physical type, a fancy one would only make your outfit look confused and anything but chic.

(2) It should preferably be **quite short**—definitely above the knee—to **take advantage of the shape of the leg in plain sight**, which is always helpful to lengthen your legs and to balance out the volume in the upper body (dark stockings allow you to wear this ensemble no matter your age).

(3) **Egg-shaped dresses** are a perfect option for those who want to **camouflage a few extra pounds in the waist and hips area**, though this may not be the most flattering choice if you are short statured. In this case it's essential to wear high heels (but *not* stilettos) and opt for a dress that is quite short in order to obtain a more proportional effect.

(4) For those who would like to look taller, another solution is to add a belt over a short, straight knit dress: a **belt** visually slims your figure, helping shape your silhouette, and for this reason it may be **a key accessory if you are below average height**.

A knit dress, though, may not be a good choice for those who—regardless of weight and body-shape—have big knees. In this case it is better to opt for a bright-colored, knee-length, sleeveless sheath dress worn over a dark turtleneck and paired with black opaque stockings so your knees remain unnoticed.

It's essential to choose good-quality fabrics and well-made cuts (even if this garment usually has a nice and easy fit). A knit dress that loses its shape after a few hours is unacceptable, as it would take class away from your look. This is not a tee that you can camouflage under a jacket or sweater; we're talking about a garment that is in fact your *entire* outfit. **The material must be impeccable and the blend faultless** (this does *not* necessarily mean expensive).

And if you want to **give verticality to your figure**, you may **add a long, shining necklace** (see chapter 27 for details), which always works to **lengthen your silhouette**. Add to this ensemble a nice pair of leather boots, and you'll get an outfit that will allow you to **feel pulled together in a totally easygoing way**. This outfit is unquestionably chic and totally suitable for many different settings.

24. Printed Skirt

The skirt is a garment that, though generally not easy to pair, **becomes a surprising staple piece in the cold season**. If properly chosen and matched, it's a versatile, timeless garment **suitable for many styles and shapes**, and it may be worn in different settings with chic results.

Though it's usually more common in the summer, a skirt becomes easier to wear when it's cooler. **When it's cold you can wear dark, opaque stockings**, which remove any drawbacks usually related to the skirt.

(1) Heavy winter stockings **don't run, they keep you warm, and they don't require shaved legs**. Therefore, in practice they're similar to trousers.

(2) Dark, heavy stockings **allow you to wear short skirts no matter what your age**, which is very good for those who would like to look taller; when there's more leg to see, this always makes your legs look longer.

(3) **If you pair dark stockings with similarly dark shoes, this removes any breakpoint between shoe and leg**, creating a long and uninterrupted vertical line that slims and lengthens your silhouette.

A printed skirt **can liven up your look (and style)**, adding energy to a dark ensemble and brightening your figure like no winter dress could ever do.

However, buying the right skirt is anything but easy. Skirts are one of the easiest—and least expensive—items to produce (trousers require much more technical expertise). Therefore, you may find in stores so many patterns that, though lovely on mannequins, may actually be quite difficult to wear.

Here are some helpful tips for a faultless choice:

- **Short A-line skirts always help your legs seem thinner and longer** (the easiest pairing is with knee-high boots, as in the picture on the right).

- **Tube skirts are to be avoided**, because they do anything but enhance your buttocks and legs (as you can see in the photo on the left).
- A **flared and knee-length design always helps make the calf look comparatively thinner**.
- For those who would like to look slimmer, remember that **carrying around too much fabric does not help**: if you want to wear patterns that are wide enough at the bottom, choose those whose wide line is given by flaring, not by curling.

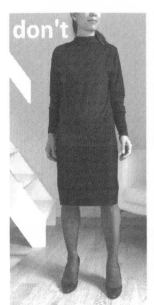 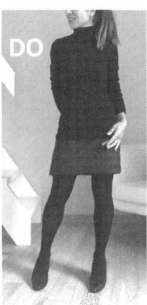 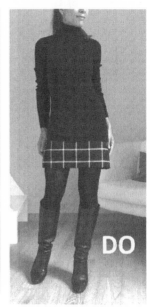

If you don't have long, lean legs, be aware that **knee-length skirts usually require heels**. Heels are particularly helpful in winter, as **they always help balance out the widening effect that heavy fabrics may have**. If you don't like high heels, opt for pretty miniskirts. Furthermore, avoid any combinations of a midlength skirt and wide ankle boots, which will end up shortening your figure.

The right skirt can also be **incredibly helpful** for those who, despite having a nice figure, complain about **a few extra pounds around the hips or thighs: a soft, flared skirt can make you gorgeous**—much more than the most cared-for trousers.

For those who would like to hide a few extra pounds around the waist but have thin legs, a good solution is a straight miniskirt paired with a long sweater. With this outfit the waist remains hidden, while your thin legs remain in sight, slimming your whole figure.

Remember that you don't need an elegant occasion to wear a skirt: you can easily wear it at work as long as the rest of your clothing is absolutely minimal. **The perfect pairing is with a dark sweater (a turtleneck is best)**, while pairings with cardigans and shirts may enlarge your body and weigh down your style.

One rule for this item is as follows: **play up your skirt and tone down everything else**.

One last thing to point out concerns the choice of **fabrics**: interestingly enough, a skirt is **exactly the opposite of other garments** in that **fancy prints can easily make a low-quality fabric almost imperceptible**, whereas a simple, straight pattern in solid color must be impeccable and of top quality to guarantee a nice outcome. A classic black tube skirt bought for $19.99 in a cheap store would look frumpy no matter what it's paired with, whereas a fancy one bought for the same price may have an outstanding outcome if properly paired with a quality turtleneck and well-made knee-high boots. This is **a great advantage for those who love eye-catching fabrics and textures**, because a skirt offers an easy way to wear them in a totally flawless way. Fancy trousers only look good on a few, and fancy shirts are difficult to wear flawlessly. Conversely, **with a fancy skirt you can please your red-carpet side or your inner princess** simply by pairing a stunning damask fabric with a simple sweater and a matching shoe, producing a fashionable outcome that will enhance your figure and style.

25. Quilted Coat with a Belt

The choice of winter outerwear is not always an easy one: most winter garments can easily widen your figure, as **heavy fabrics and padding add volume to your whole body**, making you look bulkier and—let's admit it—anything but chic. **The warmer items are often quite sporty**, whereas the more elegant and stylish ones usually are not very warm (unless you opt for a cashmere coat, but this may not be the most inexpensive option).

A lovely and interesting alternative is **a coat with a belt**: this is always a flattering solution that not only lends itself to countless pairings with different outfits but has the priceless perk of **shaping your figure, slimming and harmonizing your silhouette**.

When your outerwear is tightened at the waist by a belt, you achieve **a more sophisticated appearance**, making your waist and your whole figure look comparatively thinner and **balancing out any extra volume** caused by the heavy or quilted fabric.

This trick works with all sizes and weights, and even if you think you have a few extra pounds around your waist, the thick fabric plays down imperfections, and **the eye only perceives the hourglass figure created by the belt**, thus creating **a very chic and feminine outcome**.

Be aware, however, that your coat must have a *real* belt (made of cloth or other materials, and even if your coat doesn't come with a belt, you can always add one). **A belt creates a substantial and visible difference between your waist and your upper and lower body**, achieving a lovely and slimming effect, as you can see from the comparison between the pictures below.

Conversely, heavy overcoats that are simply close fitting around your waist may have a not-so-flattering outcome. Such a garment is generally suitable for those who are rather thin and slender, because it highlights a svelte silhouette, whereas the effect may not be the most satisfying for those who have a few extra pounds.

As for the length of this garment, you can achieve a cute and stylish outcome with a **coat that ends halfway down the leg**.

This makes **the legs look comparatively thinner, thus enhancing your whole figure**.

If you're not tall and thin, it's better to avoid long quilted coats (even if they have a belt), because in this case the belt would not be sufficient to balance out the extra volume of the padding.

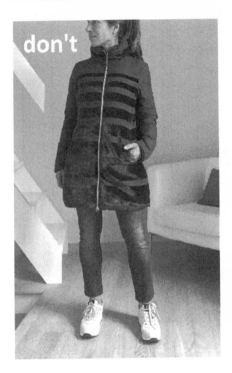 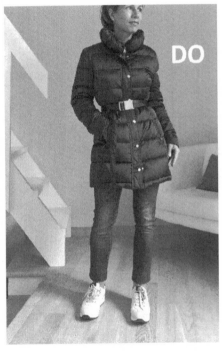

Here some other suggestions to slim your figure and obtain a chic and trendy look:

(1) **Avoid coats with zippers of contrasting colors** and, when possible, choose garments with hidden zippers. This is more chic and suggests that the garment is well made. It also produces a more flattering result, as **a zipper in plain sight widens the figure**, focusing the attention to the middle (as you can see in the picture on the left).

(2) Give preference to **belts that have a small shiny metal buckle**: it's an eye-catching element that **makes your waistline look thinner** (while driving attention away from your hips).

(3) **Raise the position of the belt itself to make your legs look longer** than they really are. This is a great slimming trick.

Here's one last trick that's always helpful for balancing out big volume in the bust area: **always pair your quilted jackets with trousers that have close-fitting legs** (but not too tight) and avoid wide-leg pants (unless you are six feet tall). Add **shoes that are at least medium heeled** (sneakers with an imperceptible wedge may also help, as you can see in the pictures above), and the outcome will be impeccable while remaining practical and easygoing.

Another lovely option is to wear **flared pants**—as long as they're *slightly* flared and close fitting around the knee—**paired with high-heeled shoes that remain hidden under the flare**: super flattering!

26. Knee-High Boots

A key item in any winter wardrobe is a pair of boots—especially for women who love wearing skirts or dresses in the cold months. When we write "boots," we don't mean *ankle* boots (which as we will see later on, are not as versatile as you might expect) but **knee-high boots**. Low-heeled or high-heeled, they **can easily give your legs a tapered shape while elongating your whole figure** and adding class to your entire look.

Knee-high boots **are indispensable for both knitted dresses and skirts**. When combined with dark, opaque stockings, they slim down the legs and the silhouette, keeping you warm and producing **a chic and stylish look** that may be suitable for many different settings.

In addition, knee-high boots **are essential even with skinny pants**, because—as you may see in the pictures below—they make your legs look more proportional instead of cutting your figure shorter, as the ankle boots may do (however, ankle boots are essential under flared pants, as we will see later).

Since knee-high boots almost completely hide the lower part of your leg, **they can be incredibly helpful for camouflaging any imperfection of the leg itself** (too thin, too full-bodied, strong calf, or not-exactly-thin ankles) **and its length** (which becomes less perceptible). These boots are very flattering when worn with overcoats that come to the knee, drawing attention to the lower part of your figure.

If you pair knee-high boots with skinny jeans and a coat with a belt worn slightly higher than your waist, your legs will look longer and slimmer, and **your whole figure will look perfectly proportional (and very sophisticated** as well).

When choosing boots that are perfect for your body type, it's essential to pay attention to a few details:

(1) One of the most important things to consider is the length of the boot leg: for those who do not have very long legs, **a boot leg may end up being too long**, which besides being uncomfortable (and *not* chic) **can make your legs look**

crooked—even if they are perfectly straight—due to the optical effect of the boot widening the outer side of your leg. The solution is to look for boots with shorter legs. This may require some time and patience, but don't worry: this is an interesting way to deepen your knowledge of what suits you more. Another option is to have your boots shortened by a good shoemaker.

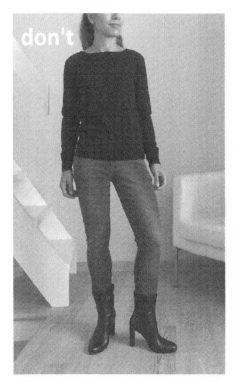
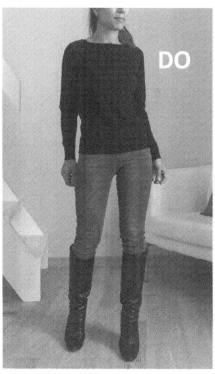

(2) Regardless of your weight and height, remember that **tucking your pants into knee-high boots is not ideal if you have short and strong thighs**. If you love this ensemble, layer it with a long knit sweater that covers your hips: this pairing guarantees a nice result, as it camouflages the actual length of your leg.

(3) If you **match knee-high boots with a flared skirt**, you'll get a timeless ensemble that can **help hide a few extra pounds in the hips area**. When wearing a short or medium-length skirt,

it's usually better to avoid any pairing with ankle boots, which can shorten your legs and enlarge your whole figure.

(4) Knee-high boots are also the perfect shoe option with a knit dress—as long as it's quite short.

Another perk of knee-high boots is that **they allow you to play with chromatic contrasts as an alternative to all-dark outfits**, which, though being widespread in the winter months, can be a little boring. If you pair light-colored trousers and knitwear with dark knee-high boots, you'll achieve a stylish look, while pairing the same ensemble with ankle boots creates a shortening effect.

Conversely, ankle boots are a must when wearing straight pants, because **knee-high boots worn under straight, close-fitting trousers only increase the circumference of your leg**, making it look more full figured (not to mention that this pairing is not elegant at all).

One last remark: knee-high boots, unless they're faux suede, must always be made with real leather. Pleather boots are anything but chic, as **fake leather used on such a large surface is clearly perceptible and will have a dowdy effect** (as opposed to pleather summer sandals, whose fake-leather straps are small enough to make the difference almost imperceptible).

If you're shopping on a budget, then it's better to opt for suede, which if well made can have a totally satisfying outcome—even if it's synthetic.

27. Necklace

As mentioned in the chapter about turtleneck sweaters, **necklaces are an extremely helpful accessory** in the winter months. They can enrich the simplest of looks, **brighten your face (and your outfit)**, and even **hide a few extra pounds**.

A necklace is a real staple accessory because it can become **an alluring touch that personalizes your whole look**, and it's versatile for many body shapes and appropriate for any setting.

A necklace draws attention to itself (and away from your hips, waist, and legs) and **visually adds a few inches to your height**.

To achieve a lovely and flattering outcome, it's necessary to pay attention to a few simple rules:

(1) Only wear one necklace at a time: **layering different necklaces can weigh down your figure**, reducing the lengthening effect that a single necklace may have.

(2) The ideal necklace should **not be too large or too elaborate**: heavy or wide necklaces can shorten your body and should be avoided if you want to obtain a slimming effect (you may still wear them in the summer or with low-cut tops).

(3) Remember that **short necklaces always highlight a short neck, making the figure appear fuller**, so be sure to consider the shape of your neck when making your choice. If you want to look slimmer, give preference to a slightly longer necklace (but not *too* long—see below).

(4) If you want to hide a few extra pounds (or look taller), **avoid too-long necklaces, which can visually lengthen the bust** and make the legs look shorter by contrast.

To achieve a slimming effect and a stylish outcome, give preference to medium-long necklaces (which naturally have a *V* shape) or to a shorter necklace with a shiny pendant in the center. The ideal size of the pendant may vary depending to your clothing choices: a **small pendant** is suitable when worn **within the neckline of an unbuttoned shirt** (picture on the right), while **a**

bigger pendant is the perfect option when you wear the necklace **over a turtleneck**, as you can see in the picture on the left.

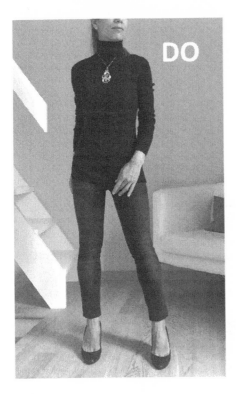
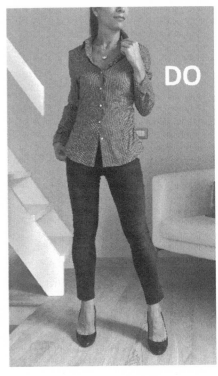

As for the materials, it's now possible to find quality costume jewelry that can produce an outstanding outcome without costing too much. You will always get a **polished and fashionable outcome** with **shining materials** that reflect light (not only metals—precious or not—but also crystal and glass). Even some **handmade necklaces made with cute stones** can be stunning and add a touch of color to a dark, monochromatic outfit.

However, even if the price is not very high, it's better—as always—to **focus on the quality of the piece and its design** rather than quantity. It's better to buy *one* fine-looking seventy-dollar necklace than ten low-quality ones for seven dollars each.

For an impeccable outcome, the metal of the necklace should match other metal details in your outfit (this is not mandatory, though: it depends on the size and position of the metal details). If the buckle of your shoes (or your belt) is gold plated, your necklace should also be gilded, whereas if your bag has huge steel details, your necklace should be silvery.

When purchasing a necklace, **you can find lovely items also in big department stores**: however, you should note that pendants in the shape of little animals, hearts, and the like are not appropriate for any woman past her twenties.

If you want to use your necklace **to add a touch of eccentricity** to your look, then **your necklace should be handcrafted**.

If you live in Europe, you should find plenty of choices: big cities and small towns alike host artisanal fairs where you can buy striking quality items with unique designs and low prices.

Vacations and trips abroad, whatever your destination, **are always good occasions to buy inimitable pieces** (as mentioned in chapter 20, the same goes for lightweight scarves and pashminas). Some costume jewelry can have poor-quality metal details, but you can always have an oxidized hook replaced with a high-quality one, and your handcrafted bone necklace will turn into a boutique piece.

If you don't live in Europe, and you're not planning a trip abroad in the next few months, **you may also buy stunning handmade necklaces online**, where you will easily find lovely items that you will never find at the mall.

Last but not least, be aware that when talking about costume jewelry, the golden rule should be **less is more**: your choices must be simple—**pay attention to the proportions**, and the result will be outstanding!

28. Leather Gloves

In winter, gloves are key accessories that protect you against low temperatures and—unexpectedly enough—**can modify the proportions of your whole figure to your advantage**.

This article, which decades ago was a fundamental component of women's clothing and had a strong seductive appeal, has over time become considered entirely unnecessary from a purely aesthetic point of view and is worn only when the weather requires it (if at all). Nevertheless, **a nice pair of gloves can be an important tool to enhance your outfit**, adding a polished touch that can enhance your chic style and **help you flatter your figure**.

Be aware, though, that when speaking of gloves, we mean *only* leather ones: gloves made of other materials (wool, fleece, or technical fabrics) may surely keep your hands warm, but they don't flatter your style (and figure) in any way. That said, you may still use gloves with wool or other materials for the inner padding in order to keep your hands warm without losing elegance.

Leather gloves are chic and sophisticated (as long as the material is quite thin), can be chosen in countless colors and patterns, and **are incredibly versatile in that they can be appropriate for many different settings and pairings**.

Thin leather gloves allow you to use your hands for anything you want: taking your keys or wallet from your bag, blowing your nose, and even answering to the phone (you may find gloves with touch-screen-friendly fingers). **Thick gloves, on the other hand, are anything but feminine, they're totally uncomfortable, and they make your hands as big as a mine worker's** while taking class away from your look (therefore, I would not recommend them for anything other than a hike up a tall mountain or a boxing match).

As for color, gloves that match your coat can produce a widening effect for your whole figure; conversely, when gloves have a color visibly different to that of your overcoat, **they can**

make your arms look shorter and your legs, in comparison, longer (as you can see from the comparison between the pictures below).

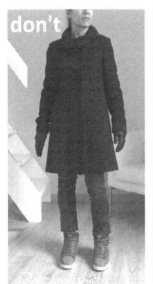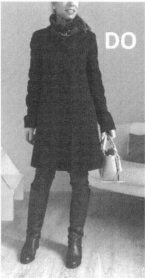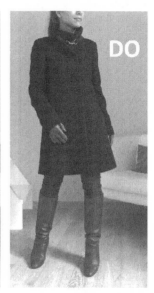

Here a few suggestions for a flawless result:

(1) To lengthen your silhouette and make the legs look longer, **the color of the gloves should contrast with the coat** (middle and right pictures). If you wear black gloves and a black coat, your arms will look visually longer and your legs comparatively shorter, as in the picture on the left. Conversely, if you wear gloves slightly lighter (or darker) than your outerwear, this will have a slimming effect, thus elongating your whole figure.

(2) Wearing gloves in a color that's different from your outerwear also has the effect of **hiding a few extra pounds in the hips area**, further contributing to visually slim your silhouette.

(3) When matching gloves to your shoes, bags, or other accessories, the easiest solution is to **pick out items that have the same type of tone (warm or cold).** For example, if your shoes are gray, blue, or taupe (cold hues), your gloves can be gray. If the accessories have warm tones (natural

leather, tan, camel, or caramel), the gloves should have a similarly warm shade (brown or any type of natural leather).

When shopping for new items, the choice may not be easy, because nice, good-quality gloves are not always cheap. But **with time and patience, you may find lovely and inexpensive articles online or on sale**.

Pay attention to the material: suede, which can be cute for brand-new gloves, will become dirty in a short time, so **it's usually better to opt for smooth leather gloves, which are also far more elegant**.

And if smooth leather is too classic for your style, you can opt for **braided leather gloves** (so chic!), which will add class and personality to your whole look in a totally easygoing way!

29. Scarf

Another fundamental accessory that goes perfectly over a sweater as well as over (or under) your outerwear is **a scarf**—not a silk or small one (already discussed earlier and more suitable for spring and autumn), but a wide and long scarf made from a warm fabric.

This article **may add vitality to an ensemble composed mainly of baseline classic pieces**, and it can **play down bold-colored overcoats** that are difficult to wear faultlessly.

A scarf allows you to easily **express your inner style and daily mood**, and it can light up both your outfit and your face.

This precious accessory also has a priceless perk: **it can visually lengthen and slim your figure**, thus flattering your silhouette in the time it takes to wrap it around your neck.

You can't take advantage of low necklines in winter (in other seasons, low necklines flatter your figure by making your bust look shorter and your legs comparatively longer). But scarves are a key accessory that can replicate the effect of low necklines in a smart and quick way.

Here a few tips to help you take full advantage of this garment and enhance your style in many different ways:

(1) **A soft and warm scarf allows you to wear low-cut garments even in winter**: if you go inside where it's warm, you can take off your scarf and take advantage of the slimming and enhancing effect of a low neckline.

(2) If you wear **a scarf in a color that contrasts with your sweater (or coat)**, you'll achieve a result visually similar to that of a low neckline, thus **making your bust look shorter** and your legs longer by comparison (as you can see in the picture in the center).

(3) Scarves are also very useful for **enhancing your face**: they allow you to **choose the colors that best suit your complexion regardless of the color of your outerwear**.

A scarf can also **bring a touch of whimsy, add a breath of energy, elevate your style**, and even reveal your personality or mood. **The same baseline outfit can look entirely different** depending on the scarf you layer over it: a colorful scarf may express your youthful spirit, a wide and soft stole can reveal your feminine side, a cashmere scarf can emphasize your inner career woman, or a trendy fur collar can make you look sultry and voluptuous.

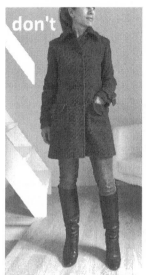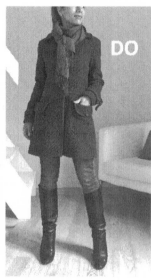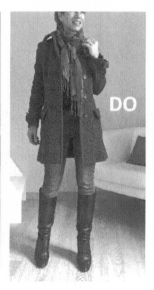

It must be said, though, that choosing the right scarf is not as easy as it may seem. The first thing to keep in mind is that you should stay away from poor-quality synthetic scarves whose only perk is a huge designer logo. Let's be clear: **for scarves, the brand is the last thing that matters**; it's better to **focus your attention on the quality of the fabric and on color**. Low-quality scarves can be spotted from a mile away (and as usual, I'm not talking about price but about material and craftsmanship). A $39.99 quilted coat bought in some inexpensive department store can look like a designer one if you add a scarf of excellent fabric, creating a trendy and stylish look, whereas a designer coat worn with a shoddy scarf will instantly turn into a cheap, low-quality garment.

As with many other accessories, the best scarf purchases are from **small or family-run businesses (you may also find them online)**. The prices are usually low enough, and quality is generally excellent. With a careful choice, though, you may also buy some quality garments in department stores (as the gray scarf in the pictures above).

Cashmere scarves can be found in knitwear factory outlets or online: remember that cashmere is produced in countless different weights, so you can also find light and delicate scarves that can be used almost all year round.

Once you have chosen your perfect scarf, **you can use it in countless ways to enhance your style and your silhouette**. For example, **you can instantly reduce the "puffy" effect** of a short quilted jacket by wearing a scarf in a color that contrasts with the jacket but is similar to the trousers: this ensemble weakens the volume effect, thus making you look proportional and stylish.

You can also create a slimming effect if you match the color of the scarf to something far from your face (shoes or bag).

In addition, **a scarf can help you to hide a poor-quality zipper** (which is sometimes the only clue that your coat is inexpensive). It can also **soften the effect that a bold color may have on your complexion**: a charcoal-gray scarf can allow you to wear a lime-green jacket that would otherwise be almost impossible to wear.

Solid-color and bicolor scarves are usually far more versatile than scarves with fancy prints. Quality is essential in this case. Avoid small prints (which don't look good on anyone) and those with too many contrasting colors. Remember that **neutral tones like the classic blue and dark gray can hide many imperfections**. If you like lively, vibrant colors, you can wear a bright-colored sweater or coat and play it down with your baseline blue (or gray) scarf for a faultless and stylish look.

For a sophisticated outcome, you may pair **shades that are similar though slightly different** (for example, a pearl-gray coat worn with a charcoal scarf or a taupe one: so chic!).

Last but not least, remember that **this accessory is essential for those with a wardrobe full of baseline interchangeable classics**: wardrobe staples are always enhanced by a well-made scarf and **may even assume a different style**. Instead of having just one dark-blue pullover in your closet, imagine if you had five. Win-win!

30. Bag in a Contrasting Color

In the cooler months, a **key element that can instantly elevate your style is a bag whose color contrasts with the colors of your outfit**.

This simple trick, as you might not expect, **can also give the appearance of a slimmer figure**. In the winter, quilted overcoats and heavy fabrics add volume to your body; if you choose a bag in a color different from the dominant color of your outfit, this will visually reduce the volume of your upper body, thus making your whole silhouette look longer and slimmer.

Conversely, **if you carry a dark bag with a similarly dark outfit, you will add volume just where you don't need it**; therefore you should avoid this ensemble if you want to look slimmer.

A light-colored or bright-colored bag can be very helpful not only in playing around with proportions but also for achieving a chic, fashionable look. **An all-dark outfit can look boring** (even if all the garments you're wearing are faultlessly paired and high quality), whereas **if you simply add a bag in a lighter (or bolder) hue, this can help you customize your outfit** with tones that are in line with your style and personality, thus creating a put-together, polished, and trendy look while enhancing your silhouette.

If your winter outfits are mainly composed of dark-colored or neutral garments, you can achieve a lovely and totally flattering outcome by adding **a light-colored or a bright-colored bag**, which can brighten a variety of looks.

If you don't like vibrant, bold colors, **you can still obtain lovely results with light-neutral hues** as long as they are visibly different from the color of your overcoat. A taupe handbag, for instance, is the perfect option for a charcoal-gray overcoat, and an oatmeal bag can look very trendy when paired with oatmeal gloves and a black jacket and pants.

If you're wearing a light-colored overcoat, then your bag should be dark colored so as not to add unnecessary volume to your figure, thus taking advantage of the slimming effect of contrasting colors.

Even though a bag is not exactly a piece of clothing, you are still carrying it on your person; if not properly paired, **it can visually enlarge your whole physique. A bag whose color contrasts with other garments** is eye-catching (it turns attention away from your hips), and it **may help hide imperfections**, boosting the slimming effect of an all-dark outfit (as you may see from the comparison between the two pictures below).

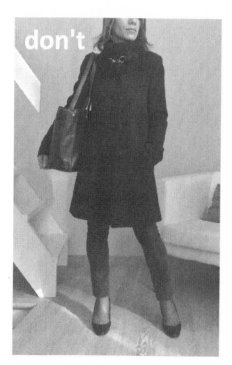 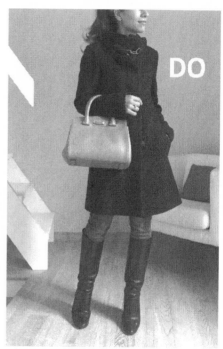

A bright-colored bag in the winter months is always an easy accessory: when your outfit is dark and monochromatic, playing around with colorful accessories is always a safe choice. Conversely, in the summer—as mentioned earlier—a bag in a bold tone can be difficult to pair faultlessly with other garments (which may be bright colored as well).

To play it safe, it's better to **combine bold accessories with an ensemble that is pretty much neutral and monochromatic**.

If you're wearing a red bag with a dark-blue coat, for example, it should be paired with dark-wash blue jeans. Avoid light blue or excessive fading.

Be careful when pairing vibrant colors with black: this ensemble can look quite outdated. It's better to pair bold colors with dark gray or with other dark neutral hues.

As for coordinating colors with other accessories, an always faultless choice is to choose items with similar shades (not identical but slightly lighter or darker). You can also obtain a very sophisticated outfit by **pairing accessories in a warm neutral shade** (for instance, tan or camel) **with an outfit in a cold neutral hue** (gray or sand beige). Similarly, a light-gray bag and gloves (cold color) can be faultlessly paired with taupe-colored garments. These combinations will always give you **a chic and sophisticated style**, thus allowing you to stand out from the crowd even when you're bundled up to the ears in your winter garments.

Now on to the subject of choosing your perfect handbag. What we mentioned in chapter 10 about leather bags is also valid for colorful or light-colored bags:

1. Your bag should preferably be **leather** (or at least **canvas**, as long as it's high quality).
2. The material must be or stiff or very soft: any in-betweens can have an unsatisfactory outcome.
3. It's essential that **metal details**—if present—are **high quality**: they must be **spotless, faultless, and sparkling**.

Just remember that **in cooler months, picking out a quality piece is particularly important for an impeccable outcome**. Carrying around a low-quality plastic bag may go unnoticed in the summer with shorts and flip-flops; however, it's anything but chic in winter.

A high-quality bag will help give you a perfect and alluring look, **boosting your style** and **revealing your taste and personality in a classy and polished way**.

PART 4

Faux Wardrobe Essentials

Faux Wardrobe Essentials

When I was eighteen and Benedetta (who besides being my coauthor is also my cousin) ten, an aunt asked her what her favorite color was. The answer, surprisingly enough, was "white and black together," which left our aunt speechless—she probably expected the answer to be the usual childish pink.

In spite of her young age, Benedetta had already fully grasped the concept of foundation pieces and baseline classics—**versatile clothing staples that never go out of style, look good on everyone, and are suitable for different settings**.

However, there are also "**faux staples**": garments that, **though traditionally considered foundation pieces, are anything but versatile** for many different reasons: because they're **only suitable for a few body shapes**, for example, or because—even if widespread—they are **very difficult to be worn and paired faultlessly**.

If a garment is not easy to match or wear, it doesn't matter how long the trends say it's essential: maybe it has interesting potential, but it *cannot* be considered a statement piece (as **is the case with the sheath dress**, which despite having great allure and many years of fashion history behind it, is nonetheless suitable for only a few body shapes and even fewer styles).

However, since **these faux staples are worn by most women**, this part of the book will provide some **suggestions to help women choose and wear these garments successfully** (or replace them with more wearable and versatile items).

The following chapters will help you **avoid the most common fashion slips**, so you can achieve a unique, outstanding look that **enhances your silhouette and boosts your style**.

31. Sheath Dress

One garment generally considered a baseline item is **the classic sheath dress**. The truth is, though, that this garment is not at all suitable for anyone: **it has low versatility** because it does not look good on any physical type and it's unsuitable for any style.

This is indeed **a quite formal garment**, and it **should only be worn by those who deeply feel it in their style**. A sheath dress may be the perfect option for **women who are traditionalists, old school, and totally self-confident** (a blend that is not very common nowadays), whereas it may not be the most appropriate choice if your style is quite informal and easygoing.

Furthermore, the classic sheath dress usually **requires a figure that's not necessarily lean but well proportioned**. For instance, a size 12 with ample breasts and wide hips can be delightfully flattered by a sheath dress, whereas a wide-busted size 4 wouldn't be. If your hips are comparatively wider than your bust (or the opposite), you'd better choose other patterns.

That said, if you look around in certain formal settings, you may notice that **many women consider a sheath dress a must for such occasions** (frequently paired with a matching jacket or blazer and black platform shoes) thus getting a look that is anything but personalized. This is too bad, because **there are so many lovely alternatives** that can be much more satisfying and suitable for formal settings—even if they have an informal character.

You don't need a "little black dress" in your wardrobe, or if you do, **it doesn't need to be a *sheath* dress**. In an ideal world, it's an exceptional item: in movies and magazines, black sheath dresses are always chic, elegant, and worn with ease, but in reality this is not the case. The sheath dress is a very difficult garment to wear, and there are countless equally chic and stylish alternatives that can be worn with a far better outcome. If you don't wear a sheath dress on a daily basis, look for another option, and you will achieve elegance and style. **On important occasions, you should only wear garments that make the most of your style** and make you feel perfectly at ease. If you are an easygoing, down-to-earth woman, put on your best jeans with a nice straight overcoat and a stylish pair of low-heeled shoes: you'll be gorgeous, and you won't look like just another chick in a not-so-flattering sheath dress.

Each of us has her own "little black dress" in the closet: it may be a nice trouser suit, **a whimsical skirt, a fancy straight overcoat, or whatever garment best fits you.** For those who love dresses—which in the warm months are always a lovely, feminine, and easy choice—it's better opt for a more informal style: for example, **a dress that's wide at the bottom may boost your physical assets while enhancing your style**, as you can see from the comparison between the pictures below. In addition to feeling at ease, you will be much more elegant than others.

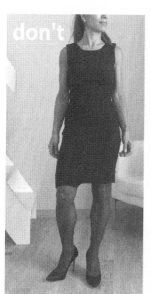 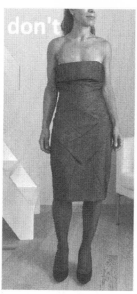 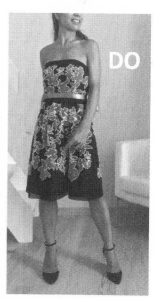

If, on the other hand, the sheath dress is part of your style (and character), be aware that some precautions are still necessary for an impeccable outcome. **To be perfect and flawless, a sheath dress should be worn *alone*** under a trench or an overcoat: this is always the easiest choice and the most slimming one. **If you want to pair your sheath dress with a jacket**, the ideal choice depends on your body shape. If you would like to look thinner or taller, it's better to **avoid pairing your dress with a matching**

jacket, because such an ensemble **may enlarge your figure**. A more flattering option is to opt instead for a long blazer (or lightweight coat) that you wear open: this will make your silhouette look thinner, producing a slimming effect for your whole figure.

Another essential detail is the quality of the fabric and cut. As this is a formal dress, **shoddy fabrics or less-than-perfect cuts are entirely forbidden**. Low-quality fabrics, which may go unnoticed with other garments, immediately reveal their poor quality on a sheath dress and make you look anything but classy. Even if you're wearing the most expensive designer shoes or your favorite Gucci handbag, a cheap, low-quality sheath dress will make your expensive accessories look fake.

As mentioned at the beginning of this chapter, **a sheath dress can enhance the figure of those with a proportional physique** (which does not necessarily mean thin). We could say it's the ideal garment for those who accumulate pounds around the whole figure: an evenly proportioned size 10 can wear this garment much better than a small-busted size 2 who gains weight only around the hips.

If you would like thinner legs, go for **a slightly flared style** (even when fashion trends want it straight), which **always has the effect of slimming the leg**. In two years fashion will have changed, and you will still be comfortable with your dress.

The ideal dress should be quite close fitting but not too tight. **It should not have any excessive design elements** (too low cut or too short), and it should not be blatantly sexy. It's up to you to play around with your feminine side by dressing it up or down with the appropriate accessories. As for the length, **the ideal sheath dress should come to the knee** (or a couple of inches higher for younger ladies). You should also avoid decorations, knots, and asymmetric cuts: this garment is stunning in a clean, linear shape; otherwise it loses all its class. With this iconic garment, two things are fundamental: the quality of the accessories and the way you wear it. With the same sheath dress, you can look like a duchess, a man-eater, a schoolgirl on her first date, a business superwoman, or an incognito princess. It's your choice!

32. Blazer

Another faux staple is **the blazer**, which is frequently worn with the sheath dress and considered a must for formal occasions. But in reality, **it doesn't always flatter your silhouette or style**.

A blazer that reaches the hips highlights what many of us usually try to hide, and **if it has a straight cut, it doesn't help boost your femininity or enhance your figure**, instead making you look boxy and much more robust than you actually are.

If you would like to look taller and slimmer, be aware that a **matching blazer and dress**, aside from creating an uninteresting outcome, produces **a shapeless effect** that's not unique or stylish (and besides, it can make you look older).

Even a blazer-shirt combination is quite difficult, because it may widen your figure.

If you love wearing blazers, **a careful choice is fundamental** for achieving a flawless outcome. Also, color combinations and proportions are crucial for this garment.

One style that is suitable for those who want to hide a few extra pounds around the thighs and hips is **a slightly flared shape that enhances the waist** for an overall slimming effect.

For those who are quite short-statured, **an interesting alternative** to the classic blazer **is a long blazer paired with close-fitting pants**: this ensemble can help you hide any imperfections around your bust and hips, making your legs seem slimmer and longer (by concealing their actual length).

For the best results, it's better to **pair a lighter-colored blazer with a darker top and pants so as to visually slim the figure**. This chromatic pairing can be applied to all kinds of jackets and coats, because it creates a vertical line that elongates your legs, slimming your whole figure (as you can see in the picture on the right). This pairing is also appropriate for wide, straight blazers, as the wide line of the jacket is balanced out by the thin silhouette of the darker top and pants. Conversely, **a blazer that's similar in color to the top is not the most flattering option**, as it may weigh your figure down. The same goes for shirt pairings, as you can see in the picture on the left.

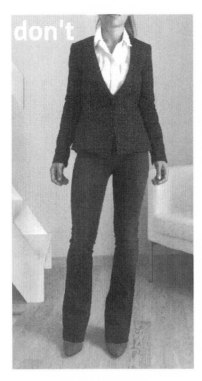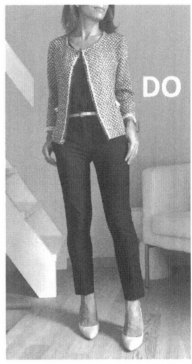

A lovely and easy alternative is **replacing the classic shirt with a soft and slightly low-cut blouse in a color similar to the pants**: this way you'll get a thin, vertical line that enhances the silhouette.

The shirt can also be replaced with a low-cut top (in spring and summer) or a turtleneck sweater (in winter), which always enhances your figure and your face. Under a formal blazer, it's often better—and it's trendier—to wear a soft top or a tee in a fine-looking fabric.

A blazer usually has **a more flattering outcome when paired with pants (even jeans), as long as they are close fitting** without being excessively tight (a combination with wider pants requires high heels if you are not very tall).

Conversely, **pairing a blazer with a skirt or a dress may look dated**, and it's not the most slimming option. As discussed previously, this ensemble has the unpleasant outcome of enlarging the whole figure due to the volume in both your upper and lower body. If it's not too cold, you may achieve lovely results wearing a nice shawl over your dress instead of a blazer (it may also be a simple scarf, if large enough and properly worn).

When wearing a blazer, **it's also essential to play down the rest of your garments**, which means wearing a smooth top and straight pants and avoiding anything that is excessively whimsical. If you want to add a feminine touch, you can opt for a silk top with a beautiful bow collar. A blazer always adds an extra breakpoint to the top and pants ensemble, and for this reason, it's essential to simplify everything you're wearing below it. This way, your blazer—instead of looking like a boring, dated garment—will allow you to express your style in chic and always stylish way.

33. Ankle Boots

In autumn and winter months, ankle boots are one of the most common shoe options. They are worn by women of all sizes and ages and paired with all kinds of garments, but in reality—contrary to the common opinion—**they are not always suitable for all body types**.

For this reason, careful consideration is a must. In a hypothetical world where we all have the legs of Gisele or Kate Moss, any combination with ankle boots and a garment randomly picked out from the wardrobe would indeed be quite good looking.

The reality, though, is a bit different: most of us have legs that are quite dissimilar to those of the top models, so the outcome is seldom the same.

If **you wear your ankle boots under flared or boot-cut trousers** (as long as they're properly hemmed—see chapter 12 for details), **you can get a faultless outcome** no matter what your body shape.

Conversely, if you wear your ankle boots *over* **your trousers or skinny jeans**, you get a result that can look good if you have thin legs (or if you can make your body look perfectly proportional with the proper pairing of garments), but **this may not be the easiest option if you would like to look slimmer or taller**. Most ankle boots **visually break the leg, making the whole figure look shorter** (whereas knee-high boots create a long, vertical line that adds length to the legs, elongating the whole figure).

Furthermore, as the styles displayed in stores are countless, **finding the most suitable style for your body type may not be that easy**. Below are a few suggestions for an impeccable yet comfortable choice.

If you want to achieve a polished and stylish look—a look that can make you chic and proportional and outlast the current trend—**it's usually better to avoid any "excessive" choice**: too squared (it's anything but feminine and chic—there is no woman in the world who can wear a shoe of this kind with grace and style), too pointy, or too bright colored.

Another style that looks good on a few women is the one with a short, wide, pleated leg: it gives you the idea of a cowboy boot that for some unknown reason has been cut shorter.

There are also styles that combine class and practicality and may enhance your legs while remaining totally wearable and easy to match. For instance, one of the most versatile styles has a two-inch block heel and a smooth, straight leg, and it makes a perfect pairing with straight pants. To get an idea of which designs are the most flattering, **just look at the classic patterns produced by top-class brands** such as Louboutin, Tod's, and Jimmy Choo. **Get inspired and look for similar (but maybe cheaper) items**—with a bit of patience, you will surely find your perfect piece.

When wearing ankle boots, **your trousers must not be too wide, and they must be properly hemmed**. A wide trouser that flutters at half length is not only totally tasteless but also has a widening effect (as on the left). The pants must follow the leg line without being too wide or too tight (the boot-cut style is usually the most flattering choice, as in the picture on the right).

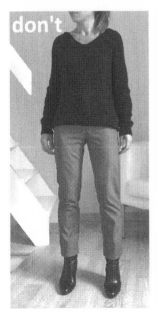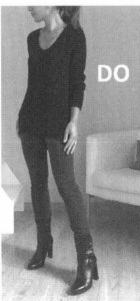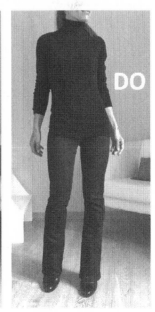

Ankle boots with a wide boot leg tend to enlarge your lower body and are therefore only suitable for those with very thin legs.

If you love to pair ankle boots with a skirt or with skinny jeans, you may opt for styles with a narrow boot leg that ends just below the calf (as in the picture in the center). **Lace-up booties are timeless and have a slimming effect**, because they don't cut your legs and create a long, vertical line that elongates your lower body (pay attention to coordinate tones, and if you're wearing a skirt, always pair it with stockings in the same color of the boot).

Don't forget that **your shoes must always be proportionate to your leg**. A properly chosen shoe should make you look slender and more graceful, so even if you have thin legs, always pay attention to the height of the heel and its width: **harmony and proportions are the keywords**, whatever your style.

If your love very high heels but are quite short-statured, you can **wear your favorite high-heeled booties under flared jeans**. This allows the heel to remain hidden, camouflaging any disproportion between your leg and the height of the heel.

Another lovely option that is as sophisticated as a pair of pumps—and is also suitable for those who do not like pumps—are **oxford heels, which are perfect in combinations with both elegant and easygoing garments**.

The essential thing, as usual, is achieving a look that is not a mere up-to-the-minute one (which will look dated in a few months) but one that **enhances your silhouette and is in harmony with your style and mood**. The results, trust me, will be impeccable.

34. Dark-Colored Handbag

An accessory that never fails in any woman's wardrobe is a black (or dark-colored) bag. Raise your hand if you have never had a bag in this color, whether it's a velvet clutch, a wide fabric bag, or a leather shopping bag.

However, as discussed earlier, **this article may be considered a staple only in a limited number of cases**. Furthermore, it usually stops being a baseline item in winter, when, interestingly enough, its use is more widespread.

In the cooler months, carrying a bag in some dark hue is quite a common choice. However, though some may assume that dark tones are the easiest option—lending themselves to pairings with many different outfits—this is not always the case. **When pairing a dark-colored handbag to a similarly dark-colored outfit**, you can get the unpleasant outcome of **widening your whole figure, adding volume and extra pounds** just where you don't need to (as in the picture on the left below). Besides, when pairing a black bag with dark garments, **the outcome is totally impersonal** and quite boring—certainly not chic.

For these reasons, a dark-colored bag is not suitable for all styles and occasions, as it has two main drawbacks: it can enlarge your figure and make your outfit look quite uninteresting.

The alternative, as mentioned in chapter 30, is **choosing a handbag whose color contrasts with the rest of the outfit**. If you opt for a bag in neutral tones like light gray or taupe, for instance, you will still have a very versatile item.

As for the dark-colored bag itself, this article may indeed be very practical thanks to the fact that it shows dirt and damage less easily than lighter-colored items. Let's see how to match it.

A well-made black bag, for example, is **very suitable for any pairings with bright-colored coats**. A few weeks ago, I noticed a girl who was wearing a stunning orange coat layered over an all-black outfit, and her stylish black bag was just perfection with this ensemble.

A black bag can also be very suitable if you want to play around with black and white. If you add a nice black bag to a bicolor top paired with a pair of straight black pants, you will get a timeless and always chic outcome.

You can also carry a dark-colored bag when wearing light-colored overcoats. When paired with light-colored garments, the dark bag **visually works the same as a light-colored one on a dark outfit**, reducing the volume of your silhouette around your hips and slimming your figure.

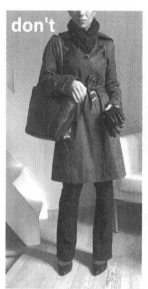 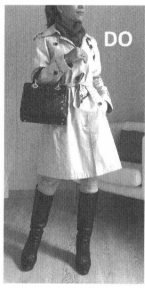 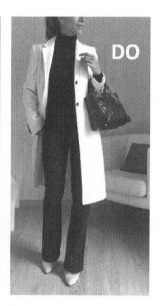

In the summer months, on the other hand, any combination of a bright-colored dress and classic black pumps paired with a black bag may look quite dated, so it's better to avoid it. Opt instead for leather-colored bags (as seen in chapter 10).

A lovely option may be a dark bag made with some unusual material or texture: for example, a braided bag or an article in some natural fiber may pop out from your outfit, adding character and personality to it.

Even for this piece, the best way to enhance your figure and style is to **play around with proportions and details**: this will always help you make the most of your physical assets and **achieve a stylish and chic look**.

35. Platform Shoes

Many women have one or more pairs of platform shoes in their closet. They're worn by heel lovers as well as by those who usually don't wear heels but want a "comfortable" option when a heel is mandatory.

However, these shoes, in spite of their (apparent) comfort, **are anything but a staple item**—not only because **they are *not* chic** but also because **they can have a totally counterproductive effect on your figure**, making you look more robust despite the fact that they are usually worn to look taller and thus, hopefully, slimmer.

Though it's totally unfair, **platform shoes may only be suitable for those who are already very tall**, as height decreases heel-to-leg disproportion and camouflages the platform, making it look lower. So if you are six feet tall (and don't care about elegance and grace), then you could wear this item; but **if you have an average leg**, be aware that **a platform does *not* enhance and does *not* stretch**—on the contrary, **it just weighs down your leg**.

Among other things, a very high platform is also a threat to your ankles, because it doesn't allow you to perceive what is under your foot until it's too late, and hitting the ground is inevitable. If your goal is to draw attention to yourself, platforms can be quite effective, yes, but if you want to sweep the man of your dreams off his feet, consider that there are more graceful ways to be seductive.

However, this ugly effect isn't present for all designs (and a slight platform can be quite comfortable); **let's see the cases in which a slight platform may be allowed (as well as a couple more reasons *not* to wear platforms)**:

(1) **A platform is *never* suitable for pumps**. The foot takes a grotesque shape and looks awfully disproportionate: you don't look taller—instead, as mentioned earlier, it looks like you're standing on a shoebox, and your legs look shorter.

(2) **The short leg effect is even greater if the shoe is dark colored** and even more so if the material is shiny.

(3) However, a platform shoe becomes **much more wearable in the form of summer sandals** with a minimalist style and in a color similar to your skin tone (as long as the platform is about half an inch).

(4) **A (slightly) thicker platform may be suitable for wedge sandals**, which if chosen in shades similar to your legs, works to lengthen the legs (see pictures on the right and in the center).

The wedge camouflages the platform better than a heel can, so pay attention and carefully choose the style of your shoes. For the best results, the wedge must be light colored (cork or rope in its natural color is perfect).

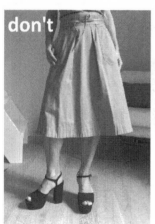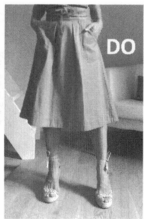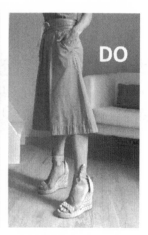

Nevertheless, be aware that **a platform shoe is *never* suitable if you want an elegant and sophisticated look** (or for formal settings), no matter its price.

Also, **avoid platforms with classic shoes styles**, such as oxfords or similar, because combining such a classic pattern with a platform is perverse.

When buying expensive designer shoes, only choose timeless styles, as they will last you years. This way, you will have a stunning piece that's appropriate for all settings, and you'll have the certainty of always making an impeccable choice. When I was in my twenties and wanted to look taller with no effort, I bought myself black platform high-heeled pumps. I then wondered *why* my legs looked shorter and more robust than when I wore cap toe ballet flats. Then I understood.

Just think about it and look in the mirror. And you will understand too.

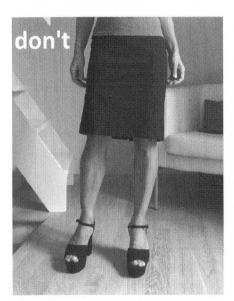 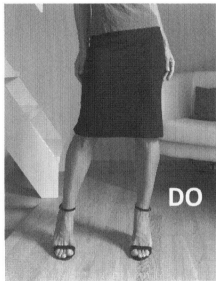

When picking out your daily outfit, be it for a business meeting, an evening out, or even a parent-teacher conference, the rule must always be taste and proportion.

Manolo Blahnik cleverly made this concept crystal clear on Vogue.com in January 2013: "I only make single-sole shoes. They transform the way a woman walks: in heavy platforms like truck drivers, in my shoes like ballerinas."

A platform gives your step a heavy, weary sound—certainly not light or graceful. **When you're approaching on platform shoes, it looks like a miner or a sumo wrestler is coming**—not a lovely, feminine girl or an alluring, chic lady: are you sure this is what you want for yourself?

Conclusion

*Style is having courage in our choices
but also the courage to say no.*
—Giorgio Armani

In these pages we have covered the main guidelines for identifying your statement pieces and pairing them so as to enhance your style while flattering your figure in multiple ways.

The next step is the practical one.

And perhaps the hardest part is to **be cautious with your purchases** and **only buy what really calls your name**: items that follow the shape of your body while hiding what you want to keep hidden—items that elevate your outfit in an instant and allow you to **achieve a unique elegance and a style (*your style!*) that is truly timeless**.

When shopping for versatile staple garments, it's essential to look for **good-quality fabrics and cuts** that combine style and taste. It's also crucial to pick out pieces that are attractive, practical, and pleasant to wear.

Your goal must be quality, not quantity.

When it comes to baseline classics, you don't need to have tons: **their versatility allows countless combinations—you can always dress these items up or down** depending on where you need to be.

Your signature jeans in a neutral shade may be worn season after season in a thousand ways and still look different every time, and the same goes for your perfect white tee or your quality leather bag.

Learn how to brighten your appearance with timeless pieces in soft, textured yarns.

Zero in on **properly chosen fabrics that can smooth bulges while visually shedding inches**. Aside from the fact that lovely materials help you achieve a chic, classy look and a unique allure, they also enhance your whole body, helping your silhouette look more toned. Low-quality materials, conversely, frequently wind up amplifying every imperfection and extra pound, highlighting faults in your figure—even where the fault doesn't exist.

My recommendation is to **change your shopping habits little by little**. Start with the search for your perfect jeans and force yourself not to buy a single garment until you've found the pair that's just perfect for you. **Focus on well-made shaping garments**, opt for clean and simple lines, and pick out structured garments that allow you to play it safe with little effort. At the same time, get rid of items that don't keep their shape anymore—those with not-so-flattering cuts or whose colors are not "you."

A little step could make a big difference, and **little by little you will declutter your closet and your whole life as well**.

This will have a positive effect on your budget and allow you to save money, space, and time.

Have fun with the search.

Make waiting become a pleasure, and **your lifestyle will benefit in every way**.

Instead of spending the whole weekend shopping for low-quality clothes that will just add clutter to your closet (and will make you forget that nice top hidden at the bottom of a drawer), dedicate the next rainy Sunday to decluttering. You don't need to overdo it: just do it little by little—a shelf at a time. Try everything on, and if you have kids (even boys!), ask for their help. Have them take photos so you can also see the rear view of your outfits: they will have much more fun than they would being dragged around shops.

And **when your craving for shopping becomes too strong**, and you still haven't found your perfect staple piece, **buy yourself a piece of underwear**. Once you've found your underwear style, it's difficult to make mistakes, so go ahead and get rid of that old, grayish, frumpy bra you keep wearing.

Don't spend money on items you know you won't wear beyond the first month.

And above all, try to **refine your taste whenever you have the chance**.

Art and nature can give you a hand, and if you look around you, **inspiration can be found in every corner**. On your next weekend off, plan a visit to a museum, an art gallery, or a craft fair (a real one with beautiful and unique handcrafted pieces). Even a visit to a botanical garden can enrich your aesthetic taste.

Focus on **finding and appreciating beauty and harmony in everything**.

Observe the clothes in paintings from Renaissance painters (you can do this online if you don't have museums close to you), admire Botticelli and Piero della Francesca, watch the films of great directors, and read fashion magazines. In short, be curious—try to educate yourself and refine your taste by studying the masterpieces in worldwide art (be it from the past or contemporary).

Take a minute to deeply enjoy the unique colors of a sunset, the nuances of the petals of a flower, and the patterns on the wings of a butterfly.

Close this book and start putting its advice into practice.

Somewhere down the line, identifying a tasteful combination or a sophisticated print from a tacky one will become natural and spontaneous. **Your style will soon become impeccable**, and you will certainly be a lady of *charme*!

About the Author

Chiara Giuliani, an architect with a passion for style and fashion, lives in Florence, Italy. After being published in academic and professional publications, in 2012 she published her first book, *La casa di charme*, a manual for making your home your own unique place, with tips to make spaces look visually bigger and more proportional. In 2016, she published her second book, *La donna di charme* (English title: *How to Become a Woman of* Charme), a manual of personal style meant to help women of all ages and body types feel more beautiful and attractive and provide them with the tools they need to build their self-confidence by enhancing their strong points. In 2017, in collaboration with her cousin Benedetta Belloni, who has been working for years in the field of custom luxury garments, Chiara founded the website www.ladonnadicharme. com and published the manual *101 Ways to Look Slimmer and Taller*, which provides useful suggestions that help flatter the figure and visually stretch out the silhouette. The book you're now holding, which develops and deepens some posts published on the website, will help you identify statement pieces that allow you to achieve a chic and stylish allure and a slender figure. It's a helpful tool for improving your image and increasing your self-esteem.

Chiara's motto comes from a famous quote:

**Beauty begins
the moment you decide
to be yourself**.
—Coco Chanel

www.ladonnadicharme.com

**Follow us on Instagram
@ladonnadicharme**

Made in the USA
Middletown, DE
03 August 2019